D0408279

$2⁰⁰

ო\ഋ൦ბ

Gardening in Clay

Gardening in Clay
Reflections on AIDS

Ronald O. Valdiserri

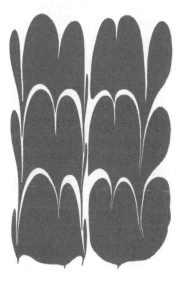

Cornell University Press
ITHACA AND LONDON

First published 1994 by Cornell University Press.

Library of Congress Cataloging-in-Publication Data
Valdiserri, Ronald O., 1951–
    Gardening in clay : reflections on AIDS / Ronald O. Valdiserri.
        p.   cm.
    ISBN 0-8014-2981-1
    1. AIDS (Disease)—Social aspects.
    2. AIDS (Disease)—Psychological aspects.   I. Title.
    RA644.A25V34   1994
    362.1'969792—dc20   93-41378

Printed in the United States of America

⊗ The paper in this book meets the minimum requirements of the American National Standard for Information Sciences—Permanence of Paper for Printed Library Materials, ANSI Z39.48-1984.

8.23.2005 Oakland

for Ray

Contents

Preface   ix

Weeds   1

Garden Memories   5

About My Brother   9

Organic Chemistry of the Spirit   13

The Epidemiology of Anger   17

Changing for the Better   22

Pieces of the Puzzle   27

Studying Disease   32

Social Mythology   36

Suffering   40

Horror Movies   43

Science Fiction   46

Patience   51

Icebergs   54

Seeing Things as They Are   58

Down There   62

Memento Mori   68

Afterlife   72

Potsherds and Dinner Plates   76

Touch and Comfort   80

Second Chances   84

Remembrance   88

Family Values   92

My Father's Bakery   96

The Language of Flowers   101

Gardening in Clay   104

Preface

I BEGAN THIS BOOK BECAUSE I WAS CONCERNED that too many of us continue to see AIDS as something that happens only to others, as a disease of "them" rather than "us." In the past I've written about AIDS from a technical perspective, primarily for researchers and specialists in the field of HIV prevention. But AIDS represents more than a rigorous challenge to our scientific skills, a complex virologic puzzle waiting for the right person to come along and crack open its secret. This disease also presents a profound challenge to our ability to understand the thoughts and feelings of people whose heritage, rearing, and life experiences may be strikingly different from ours. Exploring the social circumstances of the epidemic seemed to me to be a means of contributing to this understanding, a way to express my strong belief that AIDS is much more than just a medical or public health problem.

I didn't limit my writing to social issues that influence or arise from our society's responses to the HIV epidemic. Because my knowledge of this disease is more than professional, many of these essays are deeply personal. My twin brother, Edwin, died of HIV-related disease on November 10, 1992, before I finished this book. His illness and death and the loss of other friends and colleagues have changed my feelings about life and my notions of fulfillment. I find that I cannot see things in the same way anymore. Being a private person, expressing my grief in such a public manner hasn't been easy. But I felt to do less would have been to dishonor those whose lives have been taken by the epidemic.

In some ways *Gardening in Clay* resembles a memoir, for these essays express my own thoughts and feelings about AIDS. Yet they range widely, from teenage sexuality to life after death to Edwin and his illness. In some of them I talk about the social effects of a particular aspect of the AIDS epidemic; in others, the personal effects. They are arranged here without regard to the order in which they were written, however, and in that sense they do not form a chronicle of my life or Edwin's illness. I hope that readers will recognize in them my firm conviction that the AIDS epidemic is not a uniformly negative event. What we learn from it has the potential to make us better people and enrich our society.

I gratefully acknowledge the support and encouragement of Kathleen Kearns at Cornell University Press.

Enduring thanks go to my parents, Edwina and Ronald Valdiserri, for their faith in me and in this project.

I am especially indebted to Raymond Bedner, Jr., for his patience and understanding, and for his willingness to serve as a critical reader on the earliest versions of these essays.

And finally, special thanks go to my brother, Edwin, whose love and enthusiasm have never left me.

RONALD O. VALDISERRI
Atlanta, Georgia

Gardening in Clay

Weeds

The even mead, that erst brought sweetly forth
The freckled cowslip, burnet, and green clover,
Wanting the scythe, all uncorrected, rank,
Conceives by idleness, and nothing teems
But hateful docks, rough thistles, kecksies, burs,
Losing both beauty and utility.

WILLIAM SHAKESPEARE
Henry V

SOMETIMES IN THE SPRING, when I'm on my hands and knees among the azaleas, pulling our purslane and dandelion, I think how wonderful gardening would be if only it weren't for the weeds. Most of the time I dislike weeding, especially when I see it as a battle. Given the natural guile of the enemy, I become pessimistic, thinking that the weeds will always be one step ahead of me, that I can never defeat them. I can create huge mounds of compost from the honeysuckle vine, chickweed, and pokeberry that I remove from my woodland garden beds and still hundreds of malignant survivors will have escaped my surveillance. When my frustration grows past endurance, my war escalates to chemical weapons. I don't spray herbicides very often, though, for I'm not proud of resorting to excessive force. Weeds, it seems, are truly like troubles: prodigious, vexing, and capable of bringing out the worst in people. But like troubles, they can also coax out the best.

Sometimes, when I'm weeding, the simple action of plunging the fork into the earth, uprooting the plant, and shaking loose the soil that clings to its roots is very soothing. Plunge, pull, shake—repeated over and over, just like a mantra. On these occasions, my thoughts turn philosophical. Maybe the strong smell of the earth loosens memories from an earlier, less careworn time. Or maybe this contemplative sensibility is a by-product of repetitious action. In either case, when this mood takes over, I lose the notion that the weeds are my enemy, that their leaves and roots are acting malevolently. The weeds, I realize, are neither good nor bad; they simply exist. Gardens do not grow without weeds, and life does not unfold without misfortune. And then I think about the way my life has been touched by AIDS.

I can still remember the first time I came across a description of an unusual immune disorder in a medical journal—long before the disease even had a name. Because of my training in pathology, I was curious about this mysterious new disease. I remember feeling a ghoulish interest in an illness that could cause such tremendous, irreparable damage. Even then, before any of us knew its pathogenesis, its destructive potential was clear, and I felt, perhaps, much the same as the physicists who first glimpsed the horrendous possibilities of the atomic bomb. My scientific detachment didn't live long; AIDS soon became more than a medical curiosity for me. It began to take people I knew, friends who I had hoped would surround me all my life. Sources of comfort and understanding dried up. I started feeling like an uprooted, disenfranchised farmer of Dust Bowl days, driven from once green and fertile land and forced to migrate to unknown places.

Over that first horrible decade of its debut, AIDS managed to dissolve my sense of permanence and distort my perception of time. Before AIDS, I didn't know much about misfortune. I thought about the future primarily in terms of its potential to bring me more gratification and greater achievements. After AIDS, I understood that the future also has the power to disappoint. That knowledge has made me supremely impatient. Now it seems that nothing is quick enough for me; everything takes too long. I feel as if my internal clock has been wound so tightly that at any moment the hands might go spinning clean off the face, so rapidly are they going around and around.

AIDS changed my professional life as well. I had been content to study disease from a distance, behind a microscope. As a pathologist I thought about illness primarily as a disruption in normal physiology, and I was satisfied with the contributions I could make to patient care by diagnosing unusual tumors and peculiar lesions. But after the epidemic took hold, my interest in abnormal physiology waned. The accurate diagnosis of diseases, including AIDS, though it is an essential step in patient care, had become too passive for me, seemed to imply acceptance of the inevitability of illness. No longer satisfied with identifying disease, I wanted to learn how to prevent it from occurring. I was determined to join those who were already trying to stop the spread of the epidemic. And so, after I finished my public health degree, I left my job as a university-based pathologist to work full-time on AIDS prevention at the Centers for Disease Control and Prevention.

It would be easy to assume that the AIDS epidemic, so often associated with loss, generates nothing but sorrow in those it touches, that the personal adjustments we make are all negative. I find, on the contrary, that AIDS has helped me to clarify just what does and does not matter during our brief time in this world. The epidemic has not taken hope away from me, but it has taught me the inadequacy of looking toward the future as a means of rescue from the present. AIDS has shown me that hope is strongest in us when we seek our fulfillment in the circumstances of the present, when we refuse to defer our dreams or to accept defeat.

Sometimes when I'm working in my garden, I think about the invasiveness of weeds and disease, how they appear in the garden, in the human population, uninvited, unwelcome, capable of causing tremendous destruction if left unattended. Yes, it would be wonderful if some spectacular act of God or nature would banish AIDS from our existence. Gardeners dream that they'll awake some morning to find that the crabgrass has magically departed from the perennial beds. Weeds, though, whether real or metaphorical, will not be banished. Pain and loss are intrinsic to our existence in a temporal world. The best way to keep weeds from engulfing the garden is not to rail at the injustice of fate but to get down on our hands and knees and begin clearing them away.

Garden Memories

Though nothing can bring back the hour
Of splendour in the grass, of glory in the flower;
We will grieve not, rather find
Strength in what remains behind.

WILLIAM WORDSWORTH
"Intimations of Immortality"

I CAN'T REMEMBER A TIME when I wasn't interested in plants and gardens. Even when I was first learning to walk, I remember being awed by the neat rows of ruffled lettuce in my grandfather Vincenzo's terraced vegetable garden—especially the color. Not many shades of green can compete with the hue of well-tended leaf lettuce; the closest rivals might be the color of emerging spring grass or summer creek moss. Even as an adult, when I hear or read the word *green*, my mind returns to my grandfather's lettuce patch. Forever, those plants will be my standard of greenness.

My mother's parents lived in a shingled house in a small steel-mill town in western Pennsylvania. In the back my grandfather grew his vegetables, and in front, in the few feet between the porch and the sidewalk, my grandmother Anna grew her flowers. I was far too young to know the names of the brightly colored blooms, but zinnias and four o'clocks grown from seed were popular among the immigrant families who lived along the street. One plant in particular stays in my memory. In retrospect I think it must have been a

5

dahlia—not the dwarf, chrysanthemum-flowered kind but the spectacularly enormous "dinner plate" dahlia. Even to adults, the sheer mass of these showy flowers is impressive. Imagine their effect on a child brought face-to-face with a vividly colored flower as big as his head. I remember looking at that dahlia and actually expecting it to speak to me. After all, the flowers in the cartoons often conducted conversations among themselves and with visitors to the garden.

Those rambles in my grandparents' garden gave me my earliest appreciation of the color and form of plants. My love of fragrance I owe to Mike and Beryl, an older couple who lived in our neighborhood when I was young. About the time I turned eight, Beryl died and Mike sold the house and moved away. But while they lived there, the grounds surrounding their house were always well maintained, for they were both avid gardeners. I recall banks of flowering shrubs, a grape trellis—reputed among the older neighborhood kids to be a favorite meeting place for copperheads—and several flower beds, but what made the greatest impression on me was the densely grown circular bed of lily of the valley which surrounded the trunk of an old silver maple. Never before had I smelled anything so wonderful. By that time I was old enough to realize that many flowers have a distinctive aroma, whether sweet and pleasant as in roses or acrid and sharp as in marigolds. But in my previous experience, whatever scent a flower had was so faint that you had to get right up next to the bloom in order to smell it. The fragrance of those lilies of the valley, though, filled the air. I was fascinated that blooms so small could produce a scent so powerful and rich. Who would have guessed that ordinary flowers were capable of such feats?

There were other gardens in my childhood, and each one taught me something new. I learned how to identify plants by their leaves, how to prune roses, and how to make plants bushier by pinching back. I experimented with transplantation, moving trillium and jack-in-the-pulpit from the woods behind our house to a shady corner of the backyard. The neighbors who grew vegetables taught me that zucchini must be picked as small as possible, for age makes them fibrous and bland. Gardeners never stop learning.

My brother, too, was a gardener. By the time Edwin started his last garden he was visibly ill. Early on, the HIV-infected person can appear so utterly robust that it is difficult to imagine the seriousness of the underlying disease. Edwin had passed beyond that stage; now anyone could look at him and tell that he was sick. No longer able to work, he had moved to a smaller house. His arms and legs were as thin as sapling branches in early spring, and his feet, in his own words, had become "fiery bags of water." He seldom complained, though I know he felt poorly most of the time. Yet for an hour or so each day he would putter in his backyard, lurching from one bed to the next in his newly cultivated garden. Most garden chores were far too strenuous for him. Friends had to haul the soil supplements, and all the trees and shrubs were installed by the local nursery. But for short periods of time he could still weed, plant, and water.

He worked relentlessly to complete that garden, animated not so much by enthusiasm as by determination. I plotted his progress month by month during the growing season. Ivy and pachysandra beds followed the installation of the blue spruce and the dogwood. Next came the clematis trellis and a tight circle of mountain laurel around a bird bath, then a rudbeckia patch. On it went until most of the small plot of land surrounding his house was given over to garden.

People garden for many reasons, some practical and others aesthetic. My grandfather grew vegetables, first in Italy and later in Pennsylvania, to eat them. My grandmother raised flowers and Beryl and Mike planted lily of the valley because they gave pleasure to the senses. My brother had other reasons to garden. Although we never talked about it, I know that his last garden was a link to life at a time when so much of his attention was focused on dying. In his garden he could forget about medicines and doctor's visits. He could temporarily ignore the litany of loss being orchestrated by the virus that was slowly destroying him: less freedom to move, difficulty in remembering what he'd had for lunch the day before, embarrassment at not being able to recall the words for simple everyday objects. In his garden Edwin could think about growing and blooming. It was a place where disease could be controlled and blight prevented, where daisies and morning glories dancing in the wind could give him a sense of accomplishment, a sweetness that those of us around him, consumed by our worry and anger, simply could not provide.

Of course both of us always referred to his garden in the most ordinary terms, but we knew that it was not ordinary, that it was his last. From my brother's last garden I learned about strength and courage, about the dignity that comes from refusing to turn away from living even as death approaches.

About My Brother

How often are we to die before we go quite off this stage?
In every friend we lose a part of ourselves, and the best part.

ALEXANDER POPE
letter to Jonathan Swift, December 5, 1732

DISEASE DOES MORE THAN ROB THE BODY of function:
it also chips away at identity, at first carving off tiny slivers
and later, as the illness progresses, larger and larger chunks.
In a serious progressive illness such as AIDS, changes in
body weight, skin tone and texture, even the ability to walk
normally, document the progression of viral destruction.
The image in the mirror is no longer familiar. Parts of the
body that were once covered by lovely soft hair are now
bare. The taut and supple skin has turned flabby and sal-
low; in some instances it is covered with bulbous patches
of swollen purple, attached with the tenacity of leeches.
Strong, purposeful movement has become tentative and
tremulous. And the face, lacking its padding of subcu-
taneous fat, is suddenly dominated by lost and plaintive
eyes. This physical transfiguration signals equally profound, though less readily apparent, changes in the way the
sick person has come to think about him/herself. As the
disease advances, the person who is ill moves from inde-
pendence to dependence, from feeling carefree to being
careworn.

But it's not just the sick person who experiences the psychic metamorphosis of serious illness. Those of us who are in close emotional proximity change as well. Like subatomic particles being acted upon by some unseen energy field, we shift and reconfigure as the person we love gets sicker and sicker. The identity that we held going into the process is not the same one that we leave with at the end of it. Disease changes you. I know, it's happened to me with my brother's illness.

Humans are not solitary creatures. We were built for social interaction. Our emotions, our hopes, and our fears mean very little outside the context of our personal relationships, whether sublime or damnable. Identity is difficult to define without reference to the perceptions and expectations of those we love, our families, spouses, partners, and friends. If someone we care about thinks good things about us, we are likely to internalize those perceptions and think of ourselves as good. The expectations of those we love have great influence on our actions. So when they are profoundly changed—whether through serious illness, permanent absence, or death—we can't help but experience changes in our own identities.

I myself have always been a twin. That's how I was born and that's how I was raised. When my brother and I were infants our cribs were placed in tandem so that we could be close to each other throughout the night and in the early morning before our mother came in to feed and change us.

Our early lives were spent in each other's company, and truthfully, I have only a handful of childhood memories that don't involve Edwin. Our family tended to react to us as a pair, often calling us "Twin," instead of using our given names. As was the practice then, we were dressed in matching clothing, and because the resemblance between us was so strong, we were often mistaken for each other—even, on occasion, by our parents. Whether true or apocryphal, family lore has it that during the first three years of our lives only our sister, two years older, could tell us apart with any degree of certainty. When we were children, whatever we did was done together: building dams along the creek behind our house, getting lost together in the woods, or joining forces to devise some new form of torment for our beleaguered sister. When one of us was punished, the other would sulk as well.

During adolescence, when each of us began to lay claim to those qualities that made him unique, the physical and psychic closeness of our childhood relationship added an extra burden to the chore of becoming adult. There was a period of time when each of us viewed our twinship as a personal liability, an impediment to attaining our separate individualities. Because of this conflict, my own emotional adolescence lasted well beyond the physical transition of developing facial hair and a deeper voice. But with time and the experience of relationships beyond the twinship domain, I gained perspective on who I was, on what made me distinct. I accepted the inevitable differences between my brother and me, but I never stopped loving him, and I always took special comfort in the knowledge that he understood me better than anyone else.

Because of his illness, I have begun to think about the eventuality of no longer being a twin, no longer having someone who knows me so well that we can speak to each other using acronyms, abbreviations, and a kind of verbal shorthand—a practice dating back to our childhood. I'm angry, no doubt selfishly, at the thought of having a person who I love so much taken away from me, and I'm frightened. After a lifetime of defining myself in terms of this special bond between the two of us, I find it difficult to think about who I will be after he is gone. Will I still think of myself as a twin? I know that those who have lost their spouses or their children through death must go through similar agonies. Our roles in great part create our identities. It isn't easy to stop feeling like a husband, a wife, or a parent after years of being exactly that. The pain of losing part of one's identity must be like the pain that people feel after they have lost an arm or leg through amputation. Although the limb is gone, they continue to feel a phantom pain from where the arm or leg used to be.

Lately, my thoughts have turned to reminiscing about my childhood. The familiarity of the past is a soothing antidote to the turmoil of the present and the uncertainty of the future. One of my favorite photographs, taken on a Christmas Eve nearly four decades ago, shows my brother and me hugging each other, leaning across the ends of our respective cribs. I know that it was Christmas Eve because of our mother's compulsion to date and label each and every one of the hundreds of photographs she took of our family. Even today, nearly forty years later, I can close my eyes and remember what it felt like to hug my brother across the knobby bars of that crib. I swear I can.

Organic Chemistry of the Spirit

As far as we can discern, the sole purpose of human
existence is to kindle a light in the darkness of mere being.

CARL GUSTAV JUNG
Memories, Dreams, Reflections

I DON'T THINK THERE'S ANYTHING WORSE than having
to watch someone you love die.

The experience has taught me that what the existential
philosophers say about human existence is true: anguish is a
common emotion. But "taught" is such a puny word for the
kind of realization I'm talking about. Think of a lake full of
icy water, the kind that's so cold it takes your breath away
and makes your bones ache even after you've run out onto
the shore. Everyone who has been in before you has told
you the water is frigid, but only when you yourself plunge in
do you really understand how cruelly cold it is.

Watching my brother sicken has raised many different
emotions in me. Sometimes when I'm alone, without the
distraction of my work or other people to occupy me, I
think about Edwin and cry. Other times I'm elated to realize that I have been spared, at least for the present, from
having to confront my own inevitable death. This joyful
relief is often followed by guilt—wondering why it wasn't
me—or worse, sudden flashes of profound anxiety during
which I see life as a relentless landscape of disease and mis-

ery. The anger is there all the time, though. It isn't red-faced, hand-flailing, raging-at-the-fates anger. That at least has a beginning and an end. This anger isn't nearly so well defined or so cathartic. It's a grotesque lens, whose wavy yellow glass tints and distorts everything I see and do, all the light coming in to me and all of it passing out.

I honestly don't know what will happen to me as this drama of illness progresses to its inevitable conclusion. On the bad days I marvel that so many can ignore the depth and magnitude of the misery surrounding us, and I fear that I will never be able to regain any lightness of spirit. On the good days I like to think that I will become a better person because of this ordeal. The only certainty is that it will change me permanently.

In the adjustments individuals make as they experience life's adversities, Carl Jung and his followers found parallels to the fabled practice of alchemy. The alchemists believed that the essence of the precious was trapped within the ordinary, and they labored to find the precise process that would transmute base elements into gold. It's easy to see why Jung seized on this analogy: his life was devoted to helping people turn their painful and brutal experiences into opportunities for strengthening and purifying the spirit.

The alchemists never managed to change lead into gold, but they did pioneer the new science of chemistry. They perfected such techniques as distillation and recrystallization, which were necessary for more scientifically sound inquiries. Several centuries later, I used some of these same techniques in the organic chemistry course all premedical students were required to take. How I hated it. Every weekday morning during my sophomore year, I woke with a sense of dread as I visualized the walk from my dormitory to the building where the lectures were held. It wasn't just that the class was difficult, though surely it was. What made me so anxious was the gnawing doubt that remained with me that entire year, the uncertainty that I ever really understood what was going on in the class. I knew how to write the formulas describing halogenation and how the structure of an aldehyde differed from that of a ketone. I could even do a passable job of describing covalent bonds. But I was unable to blend these separate bits of information together in any meaningful, systematic way. I suffered through the laboratory course work and passed each of the tests, staying up all night beforehand if need be. I even managed to get a "B" at the end of the year, but my understanding of organic chemistry never progressed beyond mere memorization of facts. I failed to achieve alchemy in this academic endeavor, unable to transmute the information presented into precious knowledge.

I remember looking around the lecture hall, trying to discern if the other students were as confused as I was. Most of us, being highly competitive premeds, weren't in the habit of sharing our doubts or expressing our insecurities publicly. And so I was left with the uncomfortable suspicion that everyone else but me understood it; I was the only one who couldn't put it all together.

But this time things have to be different. The stakes are so much higher. I have to be able to understand what all this means—not just with my head but also with my soul. I could pass organic chemistry without really understanding it, and then I could go on to become a doctor and to pursue a career in public health, but I know the same isn't true for Alchemy 101. I am absolutely certain that unless I can turn this ugly and sad experience into an opportunity to grow in love and understanding, I will perish emotionally.

With all my heart, I wish that things were different, that I didn't find myself writing essays about death and loss. Since I can't change the circumstances that put me in this position, however, my next best option is to continue to search for the gold in this dross. If the one I love so much can bear the pain and infirmity of disease, then I can suffer the process of learning what it means.

The Epidemiology of Anger

Me miserable! Which way shall I fly
Infinite wrath, and infinite despair?
Which way I fly is Hell; myself am Hell;
And in the lowest deep a lower deep
Still threatening to devour me opens wide,
To which the Hell I suffer seems a Heaven.

JOHN MILTON
Paradise Lost

ONCE, WHEN I WAS DOING LIBRARY RESEARCH for a
lecture on the history of epidemics, I came across an item
about the bubonic plague in medieval Italy. The historian
was describing its sudden and profound effects on all aspects of society, including art. As an example, he cited a
little-known portrait of the Madonna in which the subject
was *in extremis,* already partially consumed by toads and
snakes.

Though the book contained no reproductions of the
painting, the image that it evoked has never left me. What
level of despair led the artist to depict the mother of Christ
not with her usual serene transcendence but as a diseased
and decomposing victim, a body, like so many others, soon
to be tossed into the gruesome anonymity of the plague pit?
The Black Death had become so pervasive that even a re-
vered symbol of Christianity could not escape its grasp.

Six centuries later, I can feel the artist's rage. I wonder

how many of his friends and family were taken by the pestilence. I imagine the helplessness he felt as he watched his town wither, realizing that his world would never again be as it was. Did the artist succumb as well, or was he one of the survivors left to cope with the pain and loss? Since 1985, when I first came upon the description of that painting, it has reminded me of the anger of people who have been personally touched by the AIDS epidemic.

It's not surprising that many people who have HIV disease are angry. Much of their anger has to do with being forced to face death decades prematurely. Nor is this a swift, painless demise; the course of AIDS is slow and debilitating, punctuated by such miserable landmarks as blindness, paralysis, and dementia. I had a friend who died several years ago after a long and painful struggle with HIV disease. Sometime after his funeral, while sorting through his possessions, his companion came across his diary. Inside in a shaking, spidery script my friend had written: "Sometimes the rage keeps me up all night."

This kind of anger is understandable. Certainly, there are reasons for hope. We enter the second decade of the epidemic with treatments, whereas ten years ago there were none, and every day brings us closer to a cure. But people who have this disease today realize that the cure may be too late for them. They're being cheated out of time, calm, and stamina by a virus that is slowly and completely destroying them from the inside out. They are angry at having to admit to themselves that twentieth-century medicine, so often seen as omnipotent, is powerless to rescue them. They hurt from the infection and from the insinuations that their circumstances are deserved, and this, too, makes them angry.

Most Americans have seen media images of ACT-UP,

the AIDS Coalition to Unleash Power, which was begun within the gay community by the playwright Larry Kramer. These men and women have adopted an angry, confrontational public persona. They have stormed economic, ecclesiastical, medical, and legislative bastions demanding that more be done to prevent and treat HIV disease. Those in the group who have HIV disease are angry for themselves, certainly, and all of them are angry because in many American cities AIDS has killed unbelievable numbers of gay men. It's not a matter of having lost one or two friends to this epidemic: many gay men have lost ten, twenty-five, even more. Entire communities have perished.

Grief is not quantifiable, and the pain that comes from losing one person we love may be no less profound than the pain that comes from losing many. Still, something unique happens when a group suffers the destruction of its members. The members begin to perceive the misfortune not just in terms of individual loss but also as a group threat. It doesn't matter that the ultimate culprit in all this is the virus: that's almost secondary. Because the group has had staggering losses, it begins to react in ways that will ensure its survival. ACT-UP's angry denunciation of society for not doing enough to stop AIDS voices a collective suspicion that society is recklessly indifferent to the epidemic or, worse, that it tacitly approves the carnage among homosexuals, drug users, and other "undesirables."

Gay men are not the only ones who see the AIDS epidemic as a threat to group survival. Long after its routes of transmission have been firmly established, the suspicion persists among some African Americans that HIV was created in the laboratory by white scientists purposely to destroy people of color. Although the majority of African Americans don't believe this story, the numbers who do are not inconsequential. To scoff at these suspicions or to view them as resulting solely from inadequate information misses the point by a mile. Consider how men, women, and children of color are overrepresented in the HIV toll. Then take a look at other health indices for racial minorities in this country. And don't forget the Tuskegee experiment, in which government researchers studied black men, without their informed consent, to learn more about the consequences of untreated syphilis. Finally, keep in mind that in our own century, and not too many years ago, the world was witness to publicly funded, nationally orchestrated genocide under Hitler's Third Reich. Although reason balks at the notion that the HIV epidemic is a racist plot, some African Americans might well have a different perspective. When we consider how the epidemic has affected their communities and take into account the historical experience of African Americans, it becomes easier to understand persistent suspicions of genocide.

Of course HIV is not premeditated genocide, either of African Americans or of gay men, but though we must reject these allegations, we ought not to ignore the feelings and the historical perspectives from which they derive. Disease is more than a personal physiological process; it is also a social experience. When groups—whether racial, ethnic, or behavioral—are unequally affected by an illness, they will begin to interpret the experience from a group perspective. And when the disease is life-threatening, group survival may come to seem even more important than individual survival. If, in addition, these groups are minorities, generally recognized as having characteristics that set them apart from the remainder of society, feelings of persecution will intensify their rage.

Among all the social issues involved in the AIDS epidemic, recognizing and accepting the anger of minority groups as legitimate might seem inconsequential. I know from working with community groups that it is not. Angry confrontation is no one's idea of enjoyment, but if the providers and planners of AIDS-related health services are not willing to listen to what a group has to say about its own perspective on the epidemic, we are telling them in effect that their feelings aren't important and their concerns don't matter. The message the group will hear is "Your survival isn't of interest to us." That kind of message can't possibly foster cooperation, and without cooperation, prevention programs can't work. We must understand that these groups, the ones who are profoundly suspicious of the motives of officialdom, are the very same ones who are being asked to work with governmental health agencies to stop the further spread of HIV in their communities.

The anger engendered by AIDS is complex. Like all human emotions, it contains both beneficial and destructive elements. In our rush to halt the spread of the virus, we must never minimize the anger of those whose lives have been affected by the epidemic, or mistakenly assume that it is solely the consequence of individual loss. Anger, too, can spread, from person to person and from one generation to the next. If we don't understand its genesis or its ability to foster mistrust, the consequences will be fatal.

Changing for the Better

Change is not made without inconvenience, even from worse to better.

RICHARD HOOKER
English Dictionary (Johnson)

Most everyone wants to be healthy. If asked point-blank, few of us would indicate a preference for illness or agree to a forfeiture of health. Yet we often do unhealthy things. We eat too much, we use alcohol and other drugs to help us cope with our sorrows and our stresses, and we have sex without taking precautions to prevent pregnancy or disease. Why do we behave this way if we really want to be healthy?

This is not a new question to those who study health or provide health services, but it has gotten increased attention in the AIDS era. Why is it that even when we know something is harmful or potentially harmful to us, we may do it anyway? To begin to unravel this paradox, keep in mind that HIV is spread through certain specific behaviors. What AIDS-prevention specialists are really trying to influence is behavior, not knowledge. Ultimately, it doesn't matter if a teenager scores a hundred on a quiz about AIDS if he believes that AIDS couldn't possibly happen to him and so he needn't bother to use a condom. I don't mean that education is worthless, only that changing behavior requires more than just supplying the reasons why it's wise to do so.

It's important not to have unrealistic expectations of what education, by itself, can do to prevent the spread of AIDS. Early in the epidemic, people were fond of saying that "education is the only vaccine we have against AIDS," but the analogy always struck me as peculiar. When we receive an influenza vaccination, we don't consciously will our immune systems to produce neutralizing antibodies: it just happens. Nor do we have to remember to use our antibodies against the influenza virus; they are activated automatically. We become fully protected against the flu without any conscious effort beyond getting the shot. Education, though, is a different kind of health intervention. We can teach people that HIV is transmitted sexually, that people are usually infected for a long time before they develop any outward signs or symptoms, and that having sex without a condom is risky, but it's possible to know all this and still have sex without taking appropriate precautions. Why?

The simple truth is that the factors that influence our behavior are extremely complicated. Accurate information is important, but not necessarily decisive. Of course we think, but we also fear, hope, trust, doubt, love, lust, and take chances. We can change our behavior, but not easily. The people who make a living studying human behavior have learned that even when the expected outcome of the change is extremely desirable—say, decreasing one's chances of contracting HIV infection by the consistent and correct use of condoms—there are likely to be substantial impediments to adopting it. The behavior of an individual is significantly affected by the behavior of the group with whom that person identifies, for example, and by that person's confidence in his or her ability to change. Behavioral scientists advise us to think about the process of changing an unhealthy behavior for a healthy one as a staircase to climb rather than a chalk line to step across. And when they explain these things, they use such words as peer group, norm, self-efficacy, and behavioral stage.

Many other people, however, even learned people, are skeptical of such notions. In my work with AIDS prevention, I have encountered researchers in basic science who consider the social sciences lightweight, chagrined legislators who expect permanent and complete behavior change after a single prevention counseling session, and technophiles who have no use for low-tech behavioral interventions that are based on the ability of the health care provider to listen, empathize, and negotiate. Those who have been trained in disciplines where phenomena are highly predictable and well explained by existing theories perhaps tend to see behavior in the same way that they would view a chemical reaction or a mathematical equation: "If we add quantity X of education of person A, the outcome will be quantity Y of healthy behavior." Others may attribute the differences between what people know and how they act to moral failings. Instead of seeing education alone as inadequate to change behavior, the moralists regard unhealthy behavior as a lack of willpower or, worse, a conscious choice of "bad" behavior over "good." According to this view, people who have been warned about AIDS but yet "choose to break the rules" by practicing unsafe behaviors have done something wrong, and aren't people who break the rules supposed to be punished?

Changing for the better is a complicated process, but there are further intricacies yet. There can be disagreement and differing perspectives on the specific actions necessary to achieve health. From the scientist's viewpoint, the healthiest behaviors are those that carry no risk. But realistically, risk-minimizing options may be easier to adopt than risk-eliminating ones. Think about a married couple where the man is infected with HIV and the woman is not. Everyone would agree that it is important to prevent the woman from becoming infected. The surest means of avoiding sexual transmission would be abstinence. But this option might not be acceptable to the couple. Instead they may decide to use condoms. Because they are minimizing their risk rather than eliminating it, does this make their behavior unhealthy? We agree that HIV infection is catastrophic, but our consensus certainly doesn't extend to means of prevention. Should we make condoms available to adolescents at school, or do we stress the importance of delaying sex? Should gay men be advised to avoid anal intercourse altogether or encouraged to think about condom-protected anal intercourse as sexually and sensually fulfilling? If we make clean needles and syringes available to drug users as a way to prevent HIV transmission, will we only encourage more people to inject drugs?

Nor is health itself a scientifically measurable quantity, a discrete chemical substance we can test for. Health has to do with how strong our hearts are and how clean our arteries, but it also embraces our sense of fulfillment and well-being, and it is enmeshed with both individual and group values. Stated most simply, what may seem healthy to some will be considered unhealthy by others.

When we talk about getting healthy or changing behavior to avoid HIV infection, it is essential to remember that the clients who come into our clinics or whom we encounter on street corners or in neighborhood gathering places must participate in decisions about their own health. Public health professionals, whether Ph.D. researchers or recovering drug users doing street outreach, should never be in the position to dictate behavior or tell people what is best for them. Instead, they should help clients clarify their own needs and develop the behavioral skills to reduce their risk of HIV infection. If we listen carefully to the people who run the risk of HIV infection, they will tell us what it is they need to live safer lives.

Pieces of the Puzzle

Not only is there but one way of doing things rightly, but there is only one way of seeing them, and that is, seeing the whole of them.

JOHN RUSKIN
The Two Paths

DURING THE MIDDLE AGES, some French scholars blamed the bubonic plague on a stupendous astrological mishap; nineteenth-century physicians believed that certain personality types were prone to develop tuberculosis. Hundreds of years of study have invalidated these erroneous beliefs about health and disease. We no longer blame the planets for epidemics, and we've known for more than a century that tuberculosis is caused by a bacterium, not by a fatalistic mental attitude. Yet one myth, which may be the most deeply rooted of all, remains—that the loss of health, especially to a preventable disease, is essentially the result of individual malfeasance.

When many of the leading causes of death in this country result from preventable diseases, it is tempting to attribute ill health to lapses in individual responsibility. After all, who doesn't know that eating too much fat will clog the coronary arteries, that cigarette smoking is dangerous, and that unprotected sex in the time of AIDS can have deadly consequences? It is tempting to believe that overweight cigarette smokers who die of heart disease and promiscuous persons who become infected with HIV are solely to blame for their circumstances.

Certainly, individual behavior is important, but it's wrong to place all the responsibility for achieving and maintaining health on the individual, while ignoring the social determinants. It is no less misguided than the belief that disease results from ominous planetary conjunctions.

Society exerts significant influences over us which ultimately affect our health. What we eat, where we live, and how we earn our living are to some extent socially dictated. Laws regulate other aspects of our behavior, especially sexual practices and drug use. Through mass communications media, we are urged toward certain consumer behaviors that affect health. And societal decisions about where and how to spend resources, especially with regard to medical care and prevention services, have profound ramifications for personal health. In these and many subtler ways, social influences are manifest in individual health.

A group of medical geographers has shown that New York City neighborhoods with a high incidence of HIV are also seriously deficient in such municipal services as garbage collection and fire protection. Does this finding mean that urban decay causes AIDS? Certainly not. That's like saying that rotten meat causes bacteria—a popular idea before we understood much about microorganisms. But it does suggest that the conditions that lead to urban decay may also help the transmission of HIV, either directly or indirectly. The economic decline of these neighborhoods, as evidenced by a tax base so weakened that it can no longer cover the basic municipal services that most of us take for granted, may mirror a more serious decline in social structures, mores, and expectations about the future. In such an environment, individual preventive action, by itself, may be inadequate to stop the AIDS epidemic because the social circumstances supporting continued transmission are much more powerful.

We live in an intricately interwoven social ecosystem, where changes in one part create disruptions in others—including health. A downturn in the economy, for example, can increase transmission of HIV in a multitude of ways. First and most obvious, economic stagnation lessens the ability of the state to offer HIV-prevention services such as HIV counseling and testing to its citizens, and those who live in communities where the risk of HIV infection is greatest often cannot afford to obtain these services through private sources. A less obvious consequence of a poor economy is increased stress on people who are out of work. During times of stress, some will turn to alcohol, and people who have sex while under the influence of alcohol or other drugs are less likely to practice safer sex. Besides, the theoretical risk of contracting HIV may appear greatly diminished in light of the immediate fears associated with unemployment: Why worry about AIDS, people may think, when I can't pay the rent? Some men and women may even be forced to supplement their incomes by bartering or selling sex. Or people who are out of work may no longer be able to afford condoms. These are just a few of the many ways that the economy can influence HIV transmission.

The individual simply cannot control all the circumstances required to achieve good health. For example, how can we blame injecting drug users for spreading HIV when we don't have adequate treatment facilities for people who want to quit? And what does responsible sexual behavior mean to a woman who sells sex to support and feed her children? Are efforts to prevent HIV in minority communities well directed if we fail to address the racism, unemployment, and drug use that plague these same communities? Culturally, we have a strong bias toward explaining failure as an individual shortcoming, and disease is no exception. Many of us have been raised with the belief that success, including success in health, is totally dependent on our individual actions. We tend to see disease as a form of personal failure. Such notions support the cruel, yet persistent attitude that there are two categories of people with HIV disease: the innocent and the guilty.

Why are we so willing to absolve society of any responsibility for maintaining our health? Why do we so eagerly take up the burden individually? Maybe we have a fear of losing control if we admit that much of what we consider individual choice is substantially affected by our economic, legislative, and social circumstances. Or maybe we don't yet have the right kind or amount of science to explain the complicated interactions between individuals and society which define health. We may know just as much about social ecology as those medieval astrologers knew about infectious diseases.

Ecology isn't only about the effect of pesticides on bird populations or logging on tropical rain forests. Ecology applies to our social environment just as much as it does to our natural one. The complex web of the food chain is not unlike the intricate connections between society and its members. When basic social structures and systems are functioning poorly, health will deteriorate too.

Illness is the result of many different elements—natural phenomena, social influences, individual behavior—acting together synergistically. HIV is often the end result of a long chain of events, some of which, when taken out of context, may appear trivial or even unrelated to the eventual outcome. Do you know the nursery rhyme describing how circumstances can cascade into catastrophe?

> *For want of a nail, the shoe was lost,*
> *for want of a shoe, the horse was lost,*
> *for want of a horse, the rider was lost,*
> *for want of a rider, the battle was lost,*
> *for want of a battle, the kingdom was lost,*
> *And all for want of a horseshoe nail.*

I've found myself mentally reciting it on more than one occasion, especially when I think about the causes of AIDS.

Studying Disease

Experience is never limited, and it is never complete; it is an immense sensibility, a kind of huge spider-web of the finest silken threads suspended in the chamber of consciousness, and catching every air-borne particle in its tissue.

HENRY JAMES
The Art of Fiction

TOWARD THE END OF MY THIRD YEAR of medical school, when most of my classmates had already decided what specialty training they would pursue after they received their medical degrees, I was still trying to make up my mind. It was not easy to choose. Pediatrics, psychiatry, and pathology all appealed to me in certain ways. One day I was certain it would be psychiatry, the next pathology, and on it went. My brother, who was attending medical school in another state, listened patiently to my vacillations during our weekly telephone conversations. Even then, before he had decided to become a psychiatrist, he had the knack of listening therapeutically. Our conversations were such a source of comfort to me that they often extended well beyond the budgeted time, eating into my grocery money and making the next week's shopping an exercise in thrift and imagination.

Eventually I chose pathology, in large part because I was afraid that if I worked in clinical medicine, I would have difficulty separating my life from my work. I suspected that

I would be unable or unwilling to put my needs above the needs of my patients and that other interests and pursuits would atrophy if I were faced with the constant, more pressing demands of the sick and dying. Being a pathologist would ensure a safe distance between me and the patient. When I left the hospital, I would not be preoccupied with worry about what was happening on the wards.

Pathology was a way for me to preserve my options. I could have the intellectual gratification of studying and diagnosing disease while retaining sufficient free time to pursue other interests—one foot in medicine and the other elsewhere. I don't mean to imply that pathology is a second-rate specialty or that pathologists are less caring than their clinical colleagues. I was simply hungry for diversity after the demands and regimentation of four years of medical school, and a clinical internship would have monopolized every moment of my time, making it all but impossible to follow other paths.

Shortly after I started my pathology training, a friend persuaded me to volunteer at a local, community-based free clinic which had sprung up in the foment of the sixties as a way to make health care more affordable and accessible. Soon I was supervising the training of volunteer counselors who diagnosed and treated clients with sexually transmitted diseases. Eventually, I became a member of the board of directors, working with other volunteer physicians to help ensure the high quality of the free services we provided.

The two worlds of health care I inhabited then were strikingly different. In the hospital, among the students and teachers of pathology, disease was an intellectual challenge, something that I had to learn to recognize through the microscopic changes it produced in human tissues. Biopsies no larger than a button were scrutinized for changes in the color and shape of nuclei, the arrangement of cells, even the presence and type of inflammatory reaction—anything that would help to explain what was happening in the patient's body. It was a separate world of specialized technology with its own arcane practices and language. Pathologists used peculiar words to communicate with one another: hematoxylin, eosin, and immunoperoxidase. And when we discussed with our colleagues, as we often did, the causes of our patients' ill health, we spoke about things we had seen in the microscopic realm.

In the other world in which I worked, in the basement of an old church, there was an entirely different culture. We never used the term *patient;* our consumers were always known as clients. We did away with the physician hierarchy of the hospital, and trained paraprofessionals worked alongside volunteer physicians, all of us dressed in jeans and other casual clothes—not a white coat in sight. Hanging prominently in the waiting room was a large piece of plywood on which was painted the Clients' Bill of Rights: the right to receive affordable and sensitive care, the right to participate in therapeutic decisions, and the right to refuse treatment. At the free clinic, disease was not an intellectual diagnostic challenge, it was a failure of the medical system, the result of inadequate preventive and primary care.

For nearly a decade I moved between these two worlds, stimulated by the dichotomy. I completed my studies in pathology, obtained my specialty certification, and became one of the teachers of pathology at the university where I'd trained. Then, because I was interested in disease as a social phenomenon, I studied for a degree in public health. Meanwhile, I remained on the board of the free clinic.

The AIDS epidemic forced a change. Pittsburgh was not in the first wave of mortality; yet before long our hospital surgeons began sending lung biopsies from the operating room requesting special tissue stains to confirm the diagnosis of *Pneumocystis carinii* pneumonia, an opportunistic infection that frequently signals the presence of AIDS. Shortly thereafter, we began a program at the free clinic to teach the men who frequented gay bathhouses what we knew about AIDS. Eventually, I joined a group of university researchers who were part of a national study to discover the cause of AIDS and to learn more about its transmission.

Slowly at first, and then more rapidly, Pittsburgh began to contribute to the national AIDS toll, and some of these weren't mere statistics but people I knew. As the epidemic unfolded in our city, I found that I couldn't stop thinking about AIDS. But my interest in the syndrome's protean microscopic manifestations and the complicated immunologic findings from our research group began to wane. The distance I had imposed between me and disease that had once been desirable, now only added to my growing anxiety. I found myself compelled to work toward prevention, toward trying to deny the virus a toehold in our community. The intellectual gratification I had derived from diagnosing disease in its myriad guises was gone, replaced by an urgent personal need to prevent its spread.

Social Mythology

ANALOGY has always seemed to me a good way to think about complicated issues; such comparisons often generate new ideas. But some of the analogies that come to mind when I think about the tangle of medical, public health, and social circumstances associated with the AIDS epidemic have been pretty strange.

It strikes me, for instance, that the virus responsible for AIDS shares several features with the serial killer. Most obvious, the two cause similar outcomes. Like the serial murderer, the retrovirus moves with consummate stealth from person to person, with disastrous results. Both have gained high visibility in the late twentieth century, though neither is new. Scientists now believe that HIV has been around for decades or longer but was never before recognized because it failed to reach epidemic proportions. And serial murder, despite the newness of the term, is not peculiar to our century. Ages past have witnessed this violent aberration.

We know that AIDS is caused by a virus that, after a long incubation period, selectively destroys essential cells in the human immune system, but without the social condi-

36

tions that promote unhealthy behavior, the epidemic can't propagate. Likewise, criminologists believe that there is an organic basis to the mental disorder that leads to serial murder, but negative social circumstances, including severe, unrelenting childhood abuse, are essential prerequisites for the development of this condition. And both diseases thrive in the shadow of the ordinary. Psychologists explain that serial killers often escape detection because of their ability to live seemingly routine lives, to pass unnoticed under the cover of normalcy. The villainous HIV also profits from its ability to remain hidden in its human host for long periods of time without generating symptoms; not realizing they're infected, people can spread the virus to others.

The shared characteristic that most concerns me about these two diseases, however, is their ability to function as modern myths about retribution, the destruction of persons as a punishment for wrongdoing. The manner in which HIV is spread, through sex and drug use, tends to reinforce such interpretations. And the fact that the victims of serial murderers are often socially disenfranchised citizens, such as prostitutes, nudges the perception that this calamity comes as a consequence of doing something that is wrong.

Today we have the scientific wherewithal to understand that disease is not divine punishment, that, as one writer put it, bad things can and do happen to good people. So why bother to seek out the mythic connotations of these diseases? Aren't the scientific and public health challenges they pose enough to ponder? Isn't it irrational to blame the persons affected by these diseases for the misfortune that has befallen them? Yet, we make a mistake if we ignore the myth, for our reactions to the complex social issues of disease are not entirely rational. Some of our perceptions derive from that shadowy and subterranean region beyond the realm of logic.

A myth is a story about societies, not individuals. Stories assume mythic proportions not because they are imaginary or fantastic but because they act as nesting places for widely held values, hopes, or fears. Stories about the AIDS epidemic, like those about serial murderers, are able to function as retribution myths because they activate subconscious fears that many of us harbor, deep-seated, irrational suspicions that something must be fundamentally wrong with people who suffer such grisly fates, that nothing like this could happen to good people like ourselves. Whether we've been touched directly by the events or know of them only through the news media, they gnaw at us with unsettling questions. Would these things happen if people were living the "right way"? What could be so wrong with our families and our ideals that such terrible things are possible? How much worse is it going to get before it stops?

Unlike other ancient beliefs that have been proven false, myths that view illness as retribution for wrongdoing have not disappeared. We've learned that malaria isn't caused by putrid air and that scrofula can't be cured by the touch of kings, but these discoveries occurred in the realm of the objective, where incremental scientific findings eventually displaced magical beliefs. The retribution myth, though, occupies the murkier domain of the subjective, where feelings are the lingua franca. Feelings may be positive or negative, admirable or contemptible, rational or irrational, but never right or wrong.

One frequent manifestation of the mythic view that diseases like AIDS are deserved rather than acquired is shame. How many years was it before families began to list AIDS as a cause of death in the obituaries? Even now, some prefer to use euphemisms such as "pneumonia" or "a long illness." Of course, these disguises are partly motivated by the desire to preserve privacy at a time when emotions are so disjointed, but at a deeper level they are often a manifestation of shame. Profound worry that if the word "AIDS" appears in print, everyone reading the obituary will wonder if the deceased was gay or a drug addict, someone who sickened and died because of "misconduct." If we're honest with ourselves, we realize that few of us are immune to these feelings.

Many whose lives have been touched by AIDS, either personally or professionally, may find this entire discussion distasteful, a denial of the individual tragedy that results each and every time someone becomes infected with HIV. But feelings don't cease to exist merely because they are irrational. In fact, when enough people share the same irrational feeling, it may take on a patina of truth. If we want to understand our reactions to AIDS, both individually and as a society, we must acknowledge human subjectivity, including mythic reactions to illness, as a potent force. Acknowledging how we feel won't make us turn our backs on science or turn us into self-righteous judges of those who are affected by AIDS. What a deep, honest look inward can do is help us keep from confusing feeling with fact.

Suffering

Knowledge by suffering entereth;
And Life is perfected by Death.

ELIZABETH BARRETT BROWNING
"A Vision of Poets"

I READ IN THE NEWSPAPER about a man whose wife and son had died of AIDS. He used to make his living as a minister but gave up his calling after his family became ill. It seems that his congregation couldn't handle "the situation" and was meager in its support and understanding. Angry and feeling unwanted, he decided to leave his church.

A woman in Chicago told me that when the organist in her church died from HIV disease, his mother was afraid to tell anyone the actual cause of death, although many already suspected it. She was fearful that if her fellow church members knew what had killed the boy, they would refuse to bury him. Instead, she told them that her son died from pneumonia.

Some religious leaders, people their followers listen to and respect, continue to describe AIDS as a righteous punishment for sinful acts. Fortunately, not all spiritual leaders follow this line of reasoning, but those who do astound me. They remind me of doctors who want to pick and choose the patients they will care for, not according to their medical training and professional responsibility, mind you, but according to personal preference and prejudice. A psychiatrist I met during my medical training, for example, told me that he wouldn't counsel clients who were obese because they made him feel uncomfortable. Even today, there are still some doctors and dentists who refuse to treat persons with HIV disease because of fear and prejudice.

I know that I am naive in my astonishment. After all, people who minister—whether they distribute medicine or the word of God—are not free of human foibles and shortcomings. Still, it shocks me when I hear about persons who are in the business of providing medical or spiritual care turning away from those who suffer from AIDS. I wonder if they aren't pushing God away, for I believe that those who suffer are closer to God's heart than the rest of us.

Undoubtedly, the way I understand suffering is influenced by my own conception of the Divinity. If I believed God's primary characteristic was omnipotence, then I might be more inclined to view suffering as a punishment. But to me, images of thunderbolts and wrathful countenances have never seemed awe-inspiring. They have always seemed like plain old human temper—raised to the nth degree. For me, what makes God God is his infinite understanding, and not just of arcane and complex facts, as if the Divinity were some kind of immense, cosmic computer. God has the ability to comprehend human feelings fully, to achieve total empathy, without the self-imposed barriers of fear, anger, and mistrust that often interfere with our human attempts to understand one another.

Because I see God as an all-knowing entity who feels and shares our pain, I don't believe that human suffering exists because of divine vengeance or spite. Nor do I believe that God enjoys our suffering. It exists because humans are neither infallible nor indestructible: we are mortal. I believe that people with serious illnesses, like AIDS, are best loved by God when they are forced to confront the painful reality that flesh was not meant to last forever. Those who are in pain come to understand the pain of others. They may not accept this knowledge with equanimity. Sometimes they are filled with bitterness even as they die. But they do understand, and to understand with one's heart the pain of others is an attribute of the Divine.

Horror Movies

Nothing ever becomes real till it is experienced—even a
proverb is no proverb to you till your life has illustrated it.

JOHN KEATS
letter to George and Georgiana Keats, March 19, 1819

IN A PARTICULAR GENRE OF HORROR MOVIE, the protagonist, an average man, slips out of ordinary events into
terrifying circumstances. He doesn't seek out this frightening encounter; his participation in it is a chance occurrence,
a random event. He may have stopped at the wrong house
to ask for directions or witnessed something that human
eyes were never meant to see. He survives his brush with the
extraordinary, and afterward the world looks the same as it
did before his encounter. Cars still stop for red lights, newspapers carry the usual quota of stories about murderers and
do-gooders, and librarians continue to insist on silence. But
the ordinary world with which he was once so familiar no
longer seems quite so real to him. He has come to realize
that the everyday events of his life can never be more than a
shroud covering over the horror he has inadvertently dis-
covered. He has seen the pods as they effortlessly assumed
the shape of their human prey, or in another variant of the
same genre, he has been pursued by malicious shadows that
are unseen to everyone but him.

The protagonist's encounter with the extraordinary results in two levels of horror: one comes from experiencing the monstrous event, and the other comes from the disbelief of the people he tries to warn. No one believes him, because the evil he describes is so unlike their everyday world and because believing him would be too terrifying. They prefer to remain oblivious to the horror that laps at their feet, blind to the evil that puddles all around, like too much rain water. The protagonist can see that they're stepping in it, maybe even sleeping under the spot where it is dripping through the ceiling, but try as he may, he can't convince others that the horror he has experienced is real.

The basic elements of most horror movie plots could be used to describe society's negative reactions to AIDS. After all, the fear of contagion and death, phobias that have persisted throughout the epidemic, are standard themes in many horror movies. Even the usual human revulsion at the sight of blood, on which horror movie directors tend to rely, has received an added boost in the era of AIDS, with the widespread knowledge that contact with HIV-infected blood can have deadly consequences. All these things are frightening, but for me at least, the most horrifying aspect of AIDS is my fear that our society will continue to underestimate the danger of the epidemic. I am afraid that not enough of us will recognize the seriousness of the threat it poses to our world, that we will not put the full weight of our societal resources into beating it.

Oh, yes, nowadays most everyone knows about AIDS. It isn't like the early years of the epidemic when there was so much inertia and denial, when some folks were arguing that the disease wouldn't spread beyond a small number of gay men and drug users. Still, too many people, like the disbelievers in a horror movie script, don't understand the potential horror of the AIDS epidemic. It isn't real to them.

They don't want to hear about the millions of families infected with HIV in the developing world or about the high rates of spread among the socially disenfranchised in our own nation. It is less frightening to believe that we're already doing everything we can to stop the spread of the virus. Like the protagonist in a horror movie script, the AIDS activists are not believed when they raise their voices in alarm because their messages are so chilling. Who wants to admit that such potential desolation surrounds us? For talking about the horror of AIDS, for trying to make it as real to us as it is to them, the AIDS activists, like the protagonist in the horror movie, are derided and scorned.

Sometimes, as the plot of the horror movie develops, the men and women living in the ordinary world eventually come to recognize the unseen menace around them. Finally, they come to believe the protagonist and join together to take action against the beast. After a difficult battle, they eventually vanquish the foe. In other scripts, the protagonist is unable to convince his neighbors and colleagues, and the monster eventually destroys him, silences the witness who has tried to warn people about what is waiting for them just within the borders of the fog or alongside a deserted country road on a dark, humid night.

I wonder which way it will end for us.

Science Fiction

Imagination and fiction make up more than three quarters of our real life.

SIMONE WEIL
Gravity and Grace

W HEN WE WERE KIDS, my brother and I used to play on a rock pile in the vacant lot behind our house. The rocks in the pile were ordinary flat brown sandstone, probably left over from facing one of the neighborhood houses. To the adults, it was just another place where we children might be found when we weren't on time for dinner, but to the children of the neighborhood, that ordinary pile of sandstone was a marvelous make-believe spaceship. Large and capable of interstellar travel, it had at least thirty or forty levels— one for the library, one for the observatory, and of course, one for the laboratory. As I recall, the ship was nuclear powered, and it had a big window in the bow out of which we watched the stars and planets whiz by.

What journeys we had on that ship. We landed on alien planets, usually populated by bloodthirsty monsters, played, with varying degrees of realism, by several of the smaller children. We had more than a few close calls. More often than not, the bay door would shut just in time, and we would take off seconds before a slimy tentacle could wrap around a crew member or a giant chela could crush one of us.

That ship and the imaginary journeys I took on it were early manifestations of my lifelong interest in science fiction. As a child I never tired of reading stories or seeing movies about the fantastic adventures that could result from improbable scientific discoveries or strange, poorly understood phenomena. When I saw the movie version of *The Time Machine,* I imagined the journeys I would have taken were I the time traveler. I would go back to ancient Egypt to confer with the pharaohs and to observe the pyramids under construction. Or I would travel into the future and return to the present with medicines that would cure fatal diseases with astonishing ease.

My interest never waned. Each time I encountered a new science fiction book or movie, I was caught up in another fantasy adventure. I saw myself as Otto Lindenbrock's nephew, descending into the crater of Sneffells Yokul on my way to the center of the earth. I wondered with apprehension if I, like so many others, would have been blinded by watching the beautiful green meteors and so become prey for the carnivorous Triffids. After reading *I, Robot* at the age of twelve, I decided to become a robopsychologist, certain that by the time I reached adulthood the amazing machines described in that book would be everyday commodities.

As I grew older, reading science fiction became less an occasion for fantasy and more an opportunity to think about sociology and psychology, two subjects that have always interested me. The authors' use of improbable scientific discoveries or peculiar natural phenomena as a springboard for exploring human emotions and social problems still holds great appeal for me. I am in awe of Ursula LeGuin's psychologically fertile comparison of waking and dreaming consciousness in *The Lathe of Heaven.* And Marge

Piercy's investigation of power and powerlessness in our society kept me thinking about *Woman on the Edge of Time* long after I had finished reading it.

Given my fondness for science fiction as a genre and my interest in its treatment of social issues, I have found myself, on occasion, thinking about the AIDS epidemic as if it were a science fiction story. The plot involves a technically advanced, well-meaning, though paternalistic alien who is responsible for creating the virus.

It begins when a brilliant and driven research scientist who is studying the genome of the human immunodeficiency virus discovers a gene segment that has a peculiar crystallography pattern. At first she suspects an equipment malfunction, but after isolating the segment, she finds that it contains an element that hasn't previously been described. It's nowhere to be found in the periodic table. After thorough investigation, she is convinced that it is like no other on earth. Fearing ridicule should she be proven wrong (her ambition is fueled by a strong core of insecurity), she keeps her research hidden from her colleagues. Then, shortly before she plans to share her final results with her fellow scientists, a mysterious laboratory fire destroys the original isolate and all her experimental records.

Several difficult months pass, during which the scientist tries, without success, to duplicate her original findings. She becomes even more uncertain of her original results, and her insecurity torments her. About this time, a peculiar man, who identifies himself as an insurance investigator, comes to ask her questions about the fire. After their initial meeting, though, the scientist is convinced that the investigator is far more interested in her lost research than he is in the catastrophe that destroyed it.

The scientist senses an intellectual depth in the insurance investigator which she finds intriguing, and so, she contrives to meet with him again. At their second meeting, when the scientist raises the possibility of arson as a cause of the laboratory fire, the investigator talks at length about the moral dilemma of using harmful means to achieve greater good. His description of human lives in terms of cost-benefit and cost-utility unsettles her. Yet, she feels a strong sympathy for him because she perceives that he, too, is tormented by insecurity.

That night she has an unusual dream. She is inside a small room with burnished green walls. Overhead shines a pale orange light. She can't see clearly because of a gritty mist filling the room, but she knows she's not alone. She can't see him very well, but she knows that the insurance investigator is there with her. When he talks to her, his voice has a high-pitched, irregular cadence that reminds her of the stridulation of insects. He tells her that he is a scientist, what she would call an economist, only his economic studies are on a planetary scale. He reveals that he, too, is plagued by doubts about his scientific abilities, that he is in the midst of a crisis about the ethics of his current research.

The investigator reveals that the manufacture and introduction of HIV into the human population is his doing. After years of careful study, following precise and exhaustive calculations, he had determined that the underprivileged and socially disenfranchised of this planet would continue to increase, and would experience progressively worse outcomes. His work predicted that the people of Earth would become increasingly polarized and splintered, global resources would be concentrated in the hands of a smaller and smaller minority while the vast majority of humans would suffer miserable poverty, preventable disease, social abandonment, and stigmatization. The investigator hypothesized that a global catastrophe such as AIDS would derail the awful outcome predicted by his data. Human leaders would be forced to confront the social injustices made manifest by the epidemic and would unite to ensure equitable distribution of the planet's resources. But now, the investigator confesses, he is not sure if he has done the right thing.

The next morning when she awakens, the scientist remembers every detail of the dream. It disturbs her greatly; she can't stop thinking about it. The story ends when the scientist calls the insurance agency to speak to the investigator, only to learn that the person she has asked for died several months ago in an automobile accident.

I suppose that others might have told the story in a different way. The alien might have been hostile, intent on crippling humankind so that he and his fiendish cohort could overrun our planet. He might have been more confident, less troubled by the ethical implications of his global experiment. Personally, I like his ambivalence and the notion of good intentions run amok. It reminds me of the real thing.

Patience

Patience, money, and time bring all things to pass.

Patience is a plaster for all sores.

Everything comes to him who waits.

PROVERBS

PATIENCE, at least according to the proverbialists, is a virtue. If we believe the old saws, those who patiently endure adversity will eventually triumph. Nothing is impossible or out of reach if one can only wait long enough.

Patience, though, is not inborn; we must learn it. Children are notoriously impatient, especially when they are anticipating pleasant things. Of course, their sense of time is different from ours. To a child of five, three months, when he or she is waiting for a birthday or a grandparent's visit, seem an eternity, for after all, ninety days represent nearly 5 percent of a five-year-old's total span of conscious existence. Three months seems a lot longer to the child than it does to his or her parents.

Children, then, perceive time differently from adults, but they also have other cognitive differences that make them impatient. Those who have studied childhood development, most notably Jean Piaget, describe the supreme egocentrism of infants and, to a lesser degree, preschool children. Young children, far more than adults, interpret external events from the perspective of their own selves, their own egos. Lacking the objective knowledge and experience of adults, young children have difficulty understanding events from perspectives other than their own. They believe that if they want or wish for something with enough conviction, it is bound to happen. It's not just naivete; it's the way they conceptualize events.

Although in adults this brand of egocentrism would be labeled unrealistic, foolish, or perhaps even delusional, in children it is both natural and endearing. Children's unwillingness to patiently accept outcomes that adults consider to be immutable is a recurrent theme in popular fiction. Remember the old MGM musicals? After all the adults had given up on a problem, the teenagers would join together and put on a show to raise the money needed to save the school or to prevent the ranch from closing. Because of their conviction, their energy, and their refusal to sit back and accept the inevitable, misfortune was averted.

Of course, life is quite different from an old MGM musical, but there are times when I think we would be better served if we acted more like children and less like adults when it comes to being patient. What's so virtuous about enduring without complaint? Why should we tolerate the intolerable? When it comes to preventing AIDS, I don't want anyone to be patient, to become so inured to the horror of HIV infection that AIDS becomes just another one of the many twentieth-century ills that we have to contend with. I don't want to count the bodies while we continue to argue about whether or not adolescents should have access to condoms, about who is going to be offended if prevention campaigns talk frankly about same-sex relationships, about whether drug users should be able to get clean needles. I want people to be impatient and pushy until this epidemic is over. I don't want us to forget, even for a moment, that AIDS is a preventable disease.

Maybe it's time for us to take a lesson from our children. Maybe we should stop thinking about the obstacles we face, about how difficult it is to solve the myriad problems associated with the AIDS epidemic, and start thinking about how we will . . . must . . . have to lick it. Other people have said the same about issues just as important and complicated as AIDS. If we can't visualize world peace or the end of global hunger, how can we ever hope to achieve them? The same is true for AIDS. If being adult means that we can't bring about the end of this epidemic because we're too busy enumerating all the barriers to stopping it, then I say let's start acting like children.

Icebergs

And as the smart ship grew in stature, grace, and hue, in
shadowy silent distance, grew the Iceberg too.

THOMAS HARDY
"The Convergence of the Twain"

The sinking of the *Titanic* is one of the most enduring stories of the twentieth century. Books have been written about that sad April night in 1912, and several movies
dramatize the events. Most recently, an undersea expedition
has produced scores of murky video images of the actual
wreckage site.

We remain fascinated with this disaster partly because of
its magnitude: over fifteen hundred lives were lost in a single
night. We are intrigued, too, by the wealth and social status
of many of the passengers. The list of the dead contains
names straight out of the social register—Astor, Guggen-
heim, and Rothschild, to name a few. But morbid interest
alone doesn't explain why this event continues to capture
the imagination eight decades later.

Some have suggested that the story holds our attention
because we have interpreted it as an allegory. The *Titanic*,
remember, in addition to being the biggest and most luxurious ocean liner of its day, was also supposed to be an
engineering marvel, touted as unsinkable. Because the ship
was constructed with discrete, watertight compartments,

54

people said that God himself couldn't sink it. Thus, its sinking on its very first voyage has been seen as a divine reprimand for overconfidence in technology and for overweening human pride.

Excessive faith in technology—in the case of the *Titanic*, the belief that its construction shielded it from the dangers of ice—may in fact have tempered the crew's judgment; in another vessel they might have slowed their speed or paid more serious heed to the ice warnings they'd received throughout the day prior to the collision. Instead, they trusted the technology, and in the end, it proved no match for the iceberg.

The AIDS disaster might be seen as a similar allegory. Scientific advances, both in the production of antibiotics and in the development of safe and effective oral contraceptives, loosened many of the strictures on sexual behavior our parents and grandparents faced. Sex wasn't necessarily more popular for our generation, but we came to rely on technology to remove, or at least minimize, the adverse consequences of sexual intercourse. Because many of the common sexually transmitted infections could be cured, post hoc, attention to preventing them waned. Why fuss with condoms when a pill or a shot would work as well? Then along came HIV, every bit as silent and deadly as that North Atlantic iceberg. Because of the long interval between infection and disease, the virus managed to spread for years before we had even an inkling of its existence. And when the crash occurred, when we realized that we were dealing with a global epidemic of deadly proportions, we also realized that we had no drugs to cure it.

There are other interesting comparisons between the sinking of the *Titanic* and the AIDS disaster. Consider how the ship's builders opted to allocate resources in fitting out their vessel. No expense was spared in making the ship luxurious. Its dining salons, lounges, and passenger rooms were smartly furnished using expensive materials, and the ship was equipped with every imaginable luxury, including a squash court, a gymnasium, a turkish bath, and the first oceangoing swimming pool. Yet, the inquiries that followed the sinking found that the complement of lifeboats on the vessel, though it met existing regulations, was inadequate for the number of passengers and crew. Even if all the lifeboats had been completely filled—and they were not—over a thousand people would have been denied escape. The *Titanic* was well equipped for every contingency but disaster.

Consider, too, how the AIDS epidemic has highlighted our society's preferences for distributing its health care resources. In cities where the epidemic is most fierce, many public hospitals have been pushed to the brink of financial disaster by having to care for large numbers of indigent AIDS patients. Because of this burden, resources that were once earmarked for preventing the infection are now being channeled into programs to treat the sick. There just doesn't seem to be enough money for both prevention and treatment. Yet, we live in a nation that routinely funds sophisticated and expensive biomedical research; where many hospitals, even those in small communities, can boast of the latest in medical equipment, capable of detecting the smallest tumor or diagnosing the most arcane complaint; where health economists have identified large numbers of elective surgical procedures that are both costly and unnecessary. In this same nation tens of millions of citizens are unable to obtain high-quality health care; vaccine-preventable diseases still thrive; drug users who seek treatment are put on waiting lists; pregnant women receive their first "prenatal" care when they enter emergency rooms in labor; and the mentally ill live on the streets in huts of cardboard and plastic. We are well equipped to provide health care services to people who are educated, motivated, and insured, but for those who do not meet these criteria—and many who are at risk for HIV or already have it do not—the health care system is ponderous, complex, and at times impregnable. We, too, are lacking in lifeboats.

When the *Titanic* sank, some saw it as a rebuke to human pride, a reminder of God's omnipotence and the frailty of human constructions. Those who had bragged that God himself couldn't sink this ship were proven spectacularly wrong. Technology was not the culprit, though; advances in science are not evil but welcome events. When technology fails us or brings about an unexpected, untoward outcome, it is usually because of our own lack of experience and judgment in applying it. Often, it is because we have unrealistic expectations; we overestimate the ability of technology to solve our problems.

The sinking of the great *Titanic* reminds me that technological advances are a means and not an end. If technology isn't being used to improve our lot, then it isn't being used properly. Technological advances by themselves won't solve our health problems, particularly if these problems relate to inequities in access to care. But perhaps the most pointed lesson of the *Titanic* is that icebergs are easier to avoid than they are to vanquish.

Seeing Things as They Are

Between the idea
and the reality
Between the motion
and the act
Falls the Shadow.

T. S. ELIOT
"The Hollow Men"

THE WORD *ideal* is used to describe everything from some people's marriages to an artist's performance of a particularly difficult work. Ideals don't exist in eternal perfection, however. They reflect social values, and social values change over time. Thus, an ideal of years past might seem ridiculous by today's standards.

During the Victorian era, for example, the ideal woman was nurturing, innately moral, and passive to a fault. She was to remain at home, rearing the children and ensuring the tranquility of the hearth. The demanding and sometimes immoral world of commerce in which men worked for wages was considered wholly inappropriate for women, who were deemed physically and emotionally unsuited to the demands of aggressive competition. Today this feminine ideal sounds like nonsense. Time and experience have shown us that human beings have multiple potentials, regardless of their sex. But to Victorian leaders, policy makers, and even the scientific community, distinguishing social roles on the basis of sex seemed not only proper but natural.

Other ideals, we hope, reflect values so timeless that we can all endorse them. No one would challenge ideals such as "everyone should be able to earn an honest living" and "no one should have to grow up hungry" as old-fashioned or outmoded. Yet, though we endorse these ideals, some of us consider it unrealistic to expect to achieve them. Jesus Christ himself told his disciples, "You will always have the poor with you." And this uncovers yet another definition of *ideal*, something that is so perfect that it can exist only in the imagination.

The distance between a real situation and the ideal we envision can sometimes be daunting. Sex provides a case in point. Ideally, it is a voluntary and completely honest interchange between two responsible people, both of whom benefit emotionally and spiritually from the physical act of love. It is a means of expressing the love between partners or spouses, a form of communion so extraordinary that poets have described it as a glimpse of the divine.

When sex approaches this ideal, it is every bit as wonderful and sacred as the poets and songwriters make it out to be, but sex has other, less transcendental incarnations. Our first attempts at sex can be puzzling, even frightening. Sometimes, people use sex merely as a means of escaping boredom or relieving tensions, especially when they have it by themselves. Others perform sexual acts without the consent of their partners, using sex as a weapon to punish, humiliate, and terrorize. Advertisers reduce sexual feelings to the level of copy, employing sexual images as social synonyms for success and acceptability. For some, sex is a simple economic interchange in which physical favors are traded for monetary gain. When we consider that our sexual feelings change as we develop physically and emotionally, it becomes apparent that real sex may often fall short of the ideal.

The distance between the real and the ideal is probably at its most glaring when we consider the emerging sexual nature of adolescents. No one likes to think about young people having sex, but they do. No one likes to hear that teenage pregnancy is a significant national health problem, but it is. Everyone would like to protect adolescents and young adults from sexually transmitted diseases, especially AIDS, but that's not possible unless we're willing to talk about both ideal and real sex.

To be beneficial, discussion of adolescent sex must accommodate the values of the people involved, both parents and children. We need to acknowledge the many problems of preadult sexual expression, instead of talking only about the rules we want to enforce. Otherwise we'll never get past the kind of standoff where some people are saying, "This shouldn't be happening," and others are quoting statistics to demonstrate that it is.

Let's begin by accepting the fact that we may not agree and then, for the sake of our children, both those who have sex and those who don't, work past conflict to reach a healthy compromise. We need to recognize that we can hold onto our ideals without ignoring reality. Ideally, we want all who are sexually active, regardless of their age, to revere sex as an exquisite form of human expression; realistically, we want them to understand that sex entails a unique set of responsibilities. School health programs should help students develop the skills they need to resist pressures that might push them into having sex before they are able to handle it responsibly. But we must also be willing to recognize that at some point, with or without parental consent, young people will explore the sexual feelings awakened by the physiological upheaval of adolescence. Sex is part of human development. When young adults do become sexually active, let's not bicker about whether or not they made the right decision. Instead, let's make sure that we help them to understand their new responsibilities to themselves and their partners, that we provide them with information and access to health services that will minimize their risks of unplanned pregnancy, AIDS, and other sexually transmitted diseases.

Those who oppose making condoms available to sexually active school students are well-motivated and caring people, but it isn't enough to uphold the ideal that sex should be delayed until people are full adults. In reality, adolescents are having sex, and while we argue, many of them suffer the consequences. Sexually transmitted viruses and bacteria don't trouble themselves over human bickering, and righteous indignation does not prevent disease.

Down There

But Love has pitched his mansion in
The place of excrement;
For nothing can be sole or whole
That has not been rent.

W. B. YEATS
"Crazy Jane Talks with the Bishop"

I ONCE ASKED MY GRANDMOTHER, out of curiosity, whether her mother had ever taken her aside and explained anything about sex to her. She thought for a while and then replied: "When I was a young girl, Nona" (as we called my great-grandmother) "took me and my sisters into the parlor and asked us to pretend that there was a large hole hidden under the carpet. 'Now, if you don't know anything about that hole and you fall into it,' she told us, 'it would be *mala fortuna* but it wouldn't be your fault. But if I told you about the hole and then you fell into it, it would be your own fault.'" My grandmother paused for a moment, then added, "Nona also told us, 'With the excuse of picking parsley, we let ourselves into the garden.'" According to my grandmother, these vague allusions were all she ever heard from her mother on the subject of sex.

Times have changed notably since my grandmother was a girl. Information about sex and sexuality is much more readily available. In fact, bookstores and libraries carry titles on human sexuality that would have been unutterable in my grandmother's day. Movies and television are more willing to recognize and portray the sexual aspects of human thought and action. Whereas married couples once had to keep to separate beds on screen to conform to the Hollywood standard of decency, now they may be shown, even on television, awakening with gentle caresses as part of a pitch to sell coffee or stepping into the shower in an ad for deodorant soap.

Comparing today's world to the one in which my grandmother was young, we could conclude that society has matured in its understanding and acceptance of human sexuality. The subject is less hidden than it was sixty-five years ago; we are more willing to acknowledge sexual feelings and situations publicly. Words such as "condom," "vaginal secretions," and "anal intercourse," which in decades past would have provoked nervous giggles or worse, are now part of the standard AIDS-prevention lexicon.

But how much progress have we really made concerning matters sexual? Sometimes I think that when it comes to understanding sex, our society has moved only from its childhood into its adolescence; we've yet to take the final step into adulthood.

Children spend a great deal of their time seeking information about the events and circumstances of their lives. Lacking the knowledge and the life experience required to develop a comprehensive world view, they are prone to overstatement, fantasy, or misperception. With adolescence and increasing knowledge comes a better perspective, but adolescents must pass through a developmental transition before acquiring the characteristics, qualities, and experiences that will define them as adults. If childhood is typified by the acquisition of knowledge, adolescence is intoxicated by experience. It's a kind of dress rehearsal, during which, under the best of circumstances, teenagers practice the skills necessary for adult survival. During this time of metamorphosis, while adult identities are being forged, adolescents are notoriously insecure about themselves, especially in relation to their peers.

The society in which my parents and grandparents were raised could be described as infantile in its social attitudes toward human sexuality. From all accounts, information about sex was hard to come by, and there were strong taboos against discussing the subject openly. Lacking both information and experience, people who grew up under these circumstances had precious little objective knowledge about their own sexual health and identities. It was as if sexual feelings were not meant to exist until after, or maybe shortly before, the marriage ceremony—arriving full-blown during the honeymoon. Physical relations between two people of the same sex were scarcely admitted to exist. Homosexuality was a topic for medical textbooks, which usually described it as a disorder of unknown etiology for which everything from castration to lobotomy was proposed as a cure. In the absence of either information about sex or social permission to discuss sexual feelings, myth and misperception flourished, as they so often do in childhood.

Now, like the adolescent who is tasting adult freedom for the first time, our society seems intoxicated by its ability to explore the sexual underpinnings of human behavior. We have ready access to the information about sex denied our parents and grandparents, and few sexual topics are taboo. Although they still exist, myth and misperception are less prevalent than in generations past. Sex can still provoke controversy, but it has lost much of its shock value. Today, Mae West wouldn't have the same trouble getting newspapers to advertise her play *Sex* as she did earlier in the century. What was once considered beyond the realm of polite conversation can now be heard regularly by the millions who view television talk shows.

Increased public awareness of human sexual behavior and knowledge about sex are partly related to the greater sexual freedom afforded by technological advances in birth control. AIDS, too, has made it necessary to learn about sexual behavior. It's hard to ignore the diversity of human sexuality in the midst of a global epidemic of a deadly sexually transmitted disease.

If we have learned to talk more openly about sex and if we know more about the diversity of human sexual behavior, however, we have yet to achieve an adult level of understanding and acceptance. Social attitudes toward homosexuality, for example, demonstrate how far we have yet to go.

Truly, we are more aware of gay men and lesbian women than our parents or grandparents were. When I asked my grandmother if she ever knew any gay people when she was a young woman, she told me no. Apparently, her only encounter with homosexuality was when one of her store clerks made a pass at her. At the time Nonnie had her hair cut very short and slicked back to the sides of her head. It was an attractive style, one that can still be seen today, nearly fifty years later, but it was rather severe. Nonnie explained that this woman, I've forgotten her name, came up to her one evening after the bakery had closed and said, "My, that's an awfully attractive haircut," and then kissed her on the lips.

"What did you do?" I asked.

"I slapped her in the face," Nonnie said.

"And then what happened?" I inquired.

"She slapped me back," Nonnie told me. And that was the end of the story.

According to my grandmother, it was only in retrospect that she recognized the sexual nature of this encounter. Such naivete would be unusual today. We do know more about gay people. In large part because of the AIDS epidemic, many Americans can now explain the mechanics of homosexual intercourse. Castration and lobotomy are no longer recommended as cures for same-sex attraction, and the American Psychiatric Association has removed homosexuality from its official list of psychopathologic diagnoses. But knowledge has not brought acceptance. Many still see homosexuality as a psychological illness or even an infection capable of being transmitted from "diseased" adults to "susceptible" youngsters. In some states laws still define homosexual behavior as criminal, and some religions continue to identify it as heinous sin, worthy of eternal damnation. For all our awareness about homosexual behavior, we still find it very difficult to see homosexuality as a legitimate part of the broad array of human emotional expression.

The way our society reacts to the subject of homosexuality reminds me of the difficulties adolescents experience in the process of acquiring adult identities. Because of the tremendous insecurity of adolescence, anyone who is different is suspect. Conformity to the norms of the group and pressure to act like one's peers often drive adolescents to do cruel and thoughtless things. In fact, one of the major psychological signs of adulthood is the ability to act autonomously, to be less restricted by the dictates of the group, to be strong in one's own sense of individuality and self.

In a society that was adult in its attitudes about homosexuality, gays wouldn't be seen as bad, merely recognized as different. People wouldn't feel personally threatened by the realization that some of their neighbors find it more physically and emotionally gratifying to form partnerships with people of the same sex. Families wouldn't think of homosexual sons and lesbian daughters as second-rate or even cause for shame. Courts wouldn't assume, ipso facto, that gay people make rotten parents. There would be no debate about whether gay men and lesbians should serve openly in the military. And legislators wouldn't pass laws that define same-sex relations as illegal. An adult society wouldn't need to enforce conformity, would permit people to differ, would ensure that all its members had an equal opportunity to grow into productive and self-fulfilled adults.

Memento Mori

*Elsewhere the dawn had come but here it was night, the
blackest and thickest of nights, though counteracted by
numerous torches and lights of every kind. They went back to
the shore, to see from nearer at hand if the sea would allow
of an attempt; it was still tumultuous and adverse. There my
uncle laid himself down on a cloth spread out for him and
twice called for cold water and drank it. Presently the flames
and the sulphureous odor heralding their approach put
everyone to flight, forcing my uncle to get up. Leaning on two
young slaves, he rose and immediately fell down dead.*

PLINY THE YOUNGER'S LETTER TO TACITUS
describing the eruption of Vesuvius, A.D. 79

In the 1860s the Italian archaeologist Giuseppe Fiorelli developed a process for making plaster casts of the corpses he encountered during his excavation of Pompeii. Actually, they weren't corpses at all but the spaces left by corpses. The volcanic ash and lava hardened to form a shell that remained intact centuries after the body inside decomposed. By injecting plaster into these cavities, Fiorelli was able to make a cast of the absent corpse as it had appeared at the moment of death.

Modern techniques employ polymer resin instead of plaster, but the effect is much the same. By using this process, archaeologists have been able to uncover important

68

information about the age, sex, and social status of Vesuvius's victims. Jewelry and other personal artifacts lying near the dead provide investigators with additional clues. Some of their stories seem obvious—the housekeeper who died clutching her master's keys or the woman whose terrified daughters clung to her skirts as they tried to flee the darkened city. Other stories remain a mystery. Why, for example, were the bejewelled remains of what was clearly a lady of position and wealth found, incongruously, in the gladiators' barracks behind Pompeii's great theater?

These poignant casts, which tell us so much about how Pompeii's unfortunate citizens died, are incapable of revealing what these people experienced in those final moments when they realized that life was leaving them. For death and dying are two separate things.

As a medical student working in a university hospital, I saw death often. Later, as a pathologist, I routinely did autopsies. During the performance of a complete autopsy, every organ is removed from the body, weighed, measured, and carefully studied for evidence of disease. Afterward, small pieces of tissue are cut away from the organs for examination under a microscope. This procedure reveals a great deal of useful medical information, not the least of which is the immediate cause of death. Working as a pathologist I got used to seeing death. I had to in order to function in an environment where some sick people could be cured of their ailments and others could not. My job was to understand the varied causes of death, to describe its antecedents to other doctors.

One might think that being so close to death, actually studying the organs of the deceased, would familiarize a person with dying. During an autopsy, though, when you hold a heart in your hands and examine it, you are looking for scar tissue or narrowed arteries, not for the love or passion that previously resided therein. And when you gently palpate the gelatinous folds of the brain's outer surface, you are searching for evidence of infarction or cerebral atrophy. A pathologist can't measure the disappointment or loss or even the relief present in that person's mind during the last days of life. The cadaver on the table, like the casts from Pompeii, is the lifeless remains of what used to be living. Although these remains can reveal a great deal about the cause of death or the chronology of disease, they don't say much about dying.

I didn't realize how little I knew about dying until my brother became ill. Before Edwin developed major symptoms of his disease, he talked a lot about what the future would bring. Later, as he got sicker, he thought ahead less often. I remember one conversation in particular. Both of us had traveled back to western Pennsylvania for a family reunion. Slipping away from the rest of the clan, we drove to our old neighborhood and parked across the street from the house we grew up in. Sitting in the car, looking up at the window of the bedroom we shared for eighteen years, I felt like someone sitting in an auditorium waiting for the play to start. It was one of those beautiful May afternoons when the wind is just warm enough to be soothing and the air is free of the stuffiness that comes later in the summer. Edwin began telling me how he wanted his assets divided after he died. I had heard his thoughtful and comprehensive plan several times before, but it got no easier to listen to this *memento mori*, this reminder of his impending death. As each item was described, my anxiety grew, until I was certain I would have to scream or push open the car door and run. Just then, Edwin let out a small laugh and told me that he didn't want to be the cause of another family story like the one about Santa Cecilia.

When my great-grandparents died, my grandmother and her siblings had a protracted quarrel about who should inherit an inexpensive framed print of Santa Cecilia. Eventually the dispute was settled, but the story entered family lore. Whenever my grandmother would bring it up, Edwin and I would glance knowingly at each other and settle back to enjoy this high Italian psychodrama. My grandmother accompanied the story with grand operatic gestures, and each time she told it, the artwork became more priceless and the acrimony more bitter. So this relatively minor event, recounted so often, took on histrionic dimensions. Edwin, in reminding me of it, understood that our laughter would defuse my fear and anxiety.

I realize now that Edwin repeated this litany of how his property would be divided as a ritual, one of several ways he tried to prepare me for his death, to get me used to the idea a little at a time. He knew that later in the course of his illness his energies would be taken up with his own more immediate needs and fears. But before that time came, he thought about the others around him.

Edwin was always the adventurous one, always the first of us to try something new. He smoked the first cigarette, challenged my parents' authority when I refused to, even lost his virginity before I did. Often I profited from his innovations, sharing in the lessons he learned from his new experiences. Even in death he was ahead of me, still willing to help me understand. Up until then I had always imagined that people who knew they were dying would be too angry and self-absorbed to do anything more than fret about their losses and agonize over their circumstances. Edwin showed me otherwise.

Afterlife

*Saith Thoth the righteous judge of the cycle of the gods great
who are in the presence of Osiris: Hear ye decision this. In
very truth is weighed the heart of Osiris, is his soul standing
as a witness for him; his sentence is right upon the scales
great. Not hath been found wickedness in him any; not hath
he wasted food offerings in the temples; not hath he done
harm in deed; not hath he let go with his mouth of evil things
whilst he was upon earth. Saith the cycle of the gods great to
Thoth dwelling in Hermopolis: Decreed is it that which
cometh forth from my mouth. True and righteous is Osiris,
the scribe Ani triumphant. Not hath he sinned, not hath he
done evil in respect of us. Let not be allowed to prevail
Amemet over him. Let there be given to him cakes, and a
coming forth in the presence of Osiris, and a field abiding in
Sekhet-hetepu like the followers of Horus.*

EGYPTIAN BOOK OF THE DEAD (The Papyrus of Ani)

OUR SPECIES' PREOCCUPATION with the possibility of
an afterlife may be the major difference between us and the
other primates, a direct consequence of our level of consciousness, our capacity to experience time longitudinally,
and our ability to anticipate our own mortality. We humans
are not the only animals on this planet possessing consciousness, but the level of our awareness permits us to see
ourselves not just in relation to our external environment

but also in the broader context of past and future. Other animals have a sense of time too, but usually in the context of well-defined cycles mediated by weather, hormones, or both. These temporal cycles are also important in our mammalian physiology, but we have the added perception of seeing time as a longitudinal process. We are aware of our own aging and ultimate mortality, and therefore, we are intensely interested in what will happen to us after we die.

Our beliefs about life after death span a wide range. The ancient Egyptians believed that the dead were conducted to the Hall of Judgment, where Maat, the goddess of truth, presided over the weighing of the heart, the seat of emotion and intellect. While the deceased looked on, his or her heart was placed on the pan of a large scale, counterbalanced by a feather, the symbol of truth. The jackal-headed Anubis tended the scales, while Thoth, the divine scribe, stood poised to record the results of the weighing ceremony. The elect, those whose hearts weighed no more than a feather, were to enjoy the rewards of Sekhet-Hetep, the Field of Peace. Those whose hearts were heavier were judged to be guilty of evil and were devoured by Amemet, a monster that was part lion, part crocodile, and part hippopotamus.

The description of the judgment ceremony comes to us from the Egyptian *Book of the Dead*, a collection of writings on the customs, prescriptions, and rituals associated with death and the afterlife. In their earliest form, portions of these texts were found written on the walls of tombs dating from nearly twenty-five hundred years before the birth of Christ. Later, they were transcribed onto papyrus scrolls. Clearly, our fascination with what happens to us after we die is at least as old as recorded human thought.

Many ideas about the afterlife are inextricably linked to

belief in a supreme being; like the Egyptians, some people see the afterlife as the kingdom of the Divinity, who grants blessed immortality as a reward to the faithful and pure of heart. Others believe in an afterlife that is independent of religion per se, a vague postmortem spiritual existence conceived as part of the natural progression of all corporeal beings, regardless of their individual religious beliefs. Still others foresee no existence at all after death.

My own ideas about an afterlife have changed over time. When I was a youngster, I thought about the afterlife primarily as a reward for good behavior. I would go to heaven if I didn't break any of the rules—at least not any of the important ones. It was like getting an "A" on a test that you had studied for all week long; you put in the time and the results were predictable. Once I got to heaven, I imagined that anything would be possible—except sin, of course. I would be able to fly around the world or become invisible, talk to famous dead people such as George Washington or Annie Oakley, and travel back in time to witness historical events that I'd only read about in books. I expected to find that things my parents or unfair earthly circumstance had denied me were commonplace in heaven. Heaven would be a real physical place, too, somewhere in the sky. It would have streets and houses and fields and vistas that would put the wonders of this earth to shame. So ordinary would sights like the Grand Canyon seem that angels wouldn't even pay much attention to them. And Niagara Falls, which I had seen on vacation, would be puny by heavenly standards. My child's mind conceived of the afterworld as a kingdom of excess, a place of unlimited experiences, where time, distance, and physical reality would no longer bind me.

As I grew older, I began to understand that the world

and its stories are a lot more complicated than anyone can really explain. I haven't lost my conviction that there is an existence beyond physical life or that the terms of that existence are influenced in some way by how we have lived as physical beings. I no longer think of heaven as a kind of grand prize for skillful game show contestants, though.

As I approach my middle years, age and circumstance have brought death nearer, made it more comprehensible. The adolescent conviction of invincibility and the bravado of early adulthood have been put away like a suit of clothing that is too tight around the middle. Now I know what it feels like to stand at an open grave and say goodbye, to throw a handful of dirt onto a box that contains the wasted remains of someone I loved. I now know the common human sorrow of outliving those I love. They can't be touched; yet I continue to feel them. No more can they speak to me; yet I still hear them. Even after they are gone, I continue to love them.

Now, in place of my childish dreams of sailing through the clouds or gazing down on the actions of the earthbound, I feel a fervent longing to be reunited with those I have loved, those who have left my life after many years of loving or too few. I have come to think of the afterlife as an opportunity to love better and longer than I have been able to do on this earth. Whether I have wings or can hear celestial choirs of harmonizing angels doesn't matter to me. Being able to love and be loved into eternity is the most wondrous thing I can imagine.

Potsherds and Dinner Plates

One does not discover new lands without consenting to lose sight of the shore for a very long time.

ANDRÉ GIDE
The Counterfeiters

I<small>N THE POPULAR MIND</small>, archaeology consists of amazing discoveries in glamorous settings—vine-shrouded Mayan temples, an Egyptian tomb filled with delicate golden treasures. The reality is considerably more prosaic. Instead of finding lost cities or uncovering storerooms of ancient riches, which are understandably rare events, most archaeologists are quite content to study more modest artifacts, including the rubble of past civilizations. From items as seemingly inconsequential as fragments of broken and discarded pottery, these scientists can tell us amazing things. Potsherds can speak to archaeologists about where and when the pottery was manufactured, about advances in ancient technology, even about changes in theological beliefs. By studying the style and geographical location of ancient pottery, scientists can trace the commercial networks of long-vanished civilizations. What a phenomenal skill it is to be able to piece together the history of a people from bits of jagged clay.

It's possible to conduct a personal archaeology of our own, I think. Our possessions also have their histories. In our cupboards are mugs and glasses and dinner plates that speak of our endings and our transitions, even changes in our beliefs. True, these pieces are not widely valued like Mycenaean ware or Attic red pottery. Probably no one else would recognize the personal epochs they mark. But they can tell stories of great individual significance. The objects on my shelves are no exception.

There, over in the corner, hardly used now, is a blue Melmac dinner plate, the sole piece that survives from the dinnerware of my early childhood. Its thick plastic is dull, knife-scarred, worn out by dinners eaten long ago. One of my earliest recollections is of how the blue plates in this multicolored collection would magically turn to green when my mother served applesauce on them. This plate reminds me of a time in my life when questions always had answers, when troubles were transitory, quickly dispatched by my parents. It is an artifact from the era of my earliest recall, a time when my brother was a part of everything that I did. Looking back to my early childhood, even as an adult, I find it difficult to separate my brother's presence and memories from my own. Was it only I who secretly hid the bread I didn't want to eat underneath the struts of the kitchen table, or was Edwin my conspirator?

Nearby is a relic from my youth: an inexpensive china gravy boat of uncertain age. This artifact marks a period of burgeoning awareness of adult interactions and expectations. As a young child, I could conceive of only two points of view: the one held by kids and the one held by grownups. It was at holiday meals, the only time the gravy boat was used, that I first began to question the dogma of adult solidarity. Aunts and uncles and cousins would sit down to dinner and discussion. I didn't understand the political or economic topics that the adults discussed following dinner, but it was plain that they differed to the point of argument on all sorts of things.

In my personal archaeology, the gravy boat also marks a

77

time of transition in my feelings about being a twin, a growing sense of how unusual the circumstances of my twinship
were. My cousins didn't seem to feel the same responsibility
toward their brothers and sisters that I did toward Edwin.
And I began to resent my own habit of considering my
brother's feelings as equal to my own, of forever needing to
be in agreement with him before I took any action.

Deep in the pantry cupboard is a set of four dinner
plates stamped with the insignia of the Strategic Air Com-
mand—now used only occasionally to prevent potted
plants from marking the furniture. Given to me by a favorite aunt, these plates were part of the mismatched set of
dinnerware that made up my very first household. When
she gave them to me, I had passed through physical adolescence; I wasn't yet completely adult, but I was in awe of the
possibilities that awaited me. I felt free—free of my parents, free of unhappy adolescent memories, free of having
to act like a twin. It was an era of emotional deregulation,
when lingering adolescent bravado buffered most of my
anxiety about the future. It seemed there would always be
time enough to accomplish what I wanted, to correct any
mistake, to make things better, to move to another job or
even to another relationship—until I got my life just the
way I wanted it.

For years I haven't used the demitasse cups that Edwin
gave me one Christmas, but I can't bring myself to get rid of
them. So they sit out of the way, on top of an old cookie tin
on a high shelf above the kitchen sink. Their provenance is
my early Middle Kingdom, the era of material and emotional prosperity following the time of the mismatched dinnerware. I was more self-possessed by then, and my re-
sentment of the emotional demands of twinship, which
had been a conspicuous landmark of my adolescence, had

eroded, leaving in its place a rich intimacy. Back then, there was nothing about me that my brother didn't know or understand. No question I had was too arcane; no concern too trivial. Earlier, I had perceived his instinctual knowledge of me as a threat; now I saw it as a wellspring. He became my dearest and truest friend.

Finally, there are the glasses, a recent acquisition. Eight polished-metal patio glasses in the bold monochromes that always attracted my brother. I found them in a cardboard box mixed in with the personal papers, correspondence, and photographs that Edwin left for me. Now, every time I open the cupboard door and see the glasses side by side, I wonder how long it will take me to completely decipher their meaning. Part of their significance is already clear. Since I've acquired them, time is no longer the limitless resource it once seemed; now it has become precious. But that is the easiest part of the text, the section I can translate without a Rosetta stone. They possess a deeper significance too, which I ponder, trying to understand the era they represent. Sometimes I think that my life's work will be to search within myself for what I once had so easily and fully in the company of my twin.

Touch and Comfort

Animals are such agreeable friends—they ask no questions,
they pass no criticisms.

GEORGE ELIOT
Mr. Gilfil's Love Story

I HAVE LIVED WITH BOTH DOGS AND CATS off and on throughout my life. People, like me, who share their lives with animals think of them as friends. Tammy, the boxer who came to live with our family when Edwin and I were in the fourth grade, soon became everyone's favorite. We admired her intelligence and relied on her loyalty, and when she died in 1969, the year my brother and I graduated from high school, all of us, including my parents, mourned her passing.

Now I live with two animals, a tabby cat and a pug dog. The tabby, Miss Puddy, is self-possessed and soigné, extremely affectionate, though somewhat demanding and prone to boredom. Having had several years of undivided attention before the dog arrived, she became accustomed to incessant compliments and frequent chin rubbings and now tends toward petulance if her demands for attention are not met immediately. Drusilla, the pug, was named after Caligula's sister. Despite the imperial provenance of her name, she could not be more down to earth, undoubtedly the most cheerful inhabitant of the house.

There is nothing I can't tell Puddy or Drusilla. Peculiar as it sounds, I sometimes wonder if they know me better than my human friends. Not in an intellectual way, of course, but in an emotional one. Even with spouses or loving partners we sometimes hesitate to share strong feelings or to express passing quirky moods. No such constraints apply with our animals. Friends are not always around when we need them, but our animals are. They see aspects of us that others may not.

Animals have an ability to bring us out of ourselves, to move us beyond our immediate problems and worries, and they react to our feelings with barometric precision, probably because of the way we communicate with them. We humans use language—either written or spoken—to convey our thoughts to one another. Animals, too, understand certain words—"sit," "heel," or "walk," for example—but human speech doesn't tell them very much. When we seek the solace and sympathy of our dogs and cats after a bitter disappointment or when we feel happy and contented, we tell them more by the way we touch them than by what we say to them.

Usually we reserve intimate touch for family members and dear friends. Under normal circumstances we wouldn't walk up to human strangers and begin to stroke and caress them, telling them how handsome they are and how much we want to befriend them, but such behavior is a typical human-animal interchange. The limited use of language brings a special sincerity to animal-human relationships. Animals, unlike humans, do not have the burden of having to react to what we say—merely to how we say it. Because so much of our communications with animals involve touch, our relationships with them are intimate.

Not coincidentally, "pet therapy" has been advocated for geriatric patients, autistic children, and people with AIDS. All these people benefit from human-animal interaction, and some studies indicate that elderly people who live alone may live longer and stay healthier when they share their lives with animals. I can testify that they help with grief.

My first loss to AIDS was Martin, who had been my close friend, and Edwin's, since college. Shortly after I returned from his funeral, I had to attend an important social function at my university. I wasn't in the mood to socialize and make small talk with lots of people who knew me very well professionally and not at all personally. I wanted to stay at home, nursing my sorrow, reading through the letters and postcards that I had received from Martin over the twenty years of our friendship. But I was expected to receive an award at the event, and my absence would have been awkward to explain, since none of my academic colleagues knew of my recent loss.

Never before as an adult had I been through the experience of death. I was confused and angry, but I didn't want to call Edwin, who had flown to the funeral in Florida with me and had since returned home. He had enough to cope with, knowing that the same fate awaited him. I couldn't ask him to commiserate with me when I knew how frightening the funeral must have been for him. There were others I could have turned to, but pride and my sense of privacy kept me from acknowledging my sorrow. As I sat drinking vodka and thinking about how much I would miss Martin in the years ahead, I turned to Puddy for comfort. Holding her and stroking her fur, feeling her purr beneath my hands somehow diluted the awful images that shot through my mind. I told her things that I wasn't ready to admit to anyone else. How seeing Martin's sister mourn the loss of her beloved brother generated a nauseating dread when I thought about Edwin's illness. Of course, Puddy couldn't answer me—but she didn't have to. Instead, she gave me the opportunity to express my secret fears. Afterward, I was able to leave the house and do what was expected of me.

Second Chances

You've been given a great gift, George. A chance to see what the world would be like without you.

IT'S A WONDERFUL LIFE

STARTING ABOUT THANKSGIVING and throughout the holiday season until New Year's Day, television viewers have no trouble finding opportunities to view Frank Capra's sentimental 1946 film *It's a Wonderful Life*. In the well-known story a small-town family man's despair is transformed into hope through the divinely orchestrated experience of witnessing what life would have been like had he never been born. Some critics dismiss the movie as maudlin; others consider it a Christmas classic on a par with *A Christmas Carol*, Charles Dickens's tale of personal transformation and redemption. However uneven the critical response, though, it's difficult to ignore the movie's continued popularity nearly fifty years after its premier.

Nostalgia accounts for some of the movie's staying power. Americans are particularly sentimental about idyllic depictions of small-town life. But the film also touches on deeper emotions, and two themes, in particular, are responsible for its consistent appeal: first, the idea that human accomplishments of lasting significance are not always the spectacular deeds of the powerful few but often the everyday actions of ordinary people and, second, the film's conclusion that defeat is not the inevitable outcome of despair.

84

Because he never achieved the goals he had set for himself as a young man, George Bailey thinks that his life is a failure. Only when he has an opportunity to see what Bedford Falls would be like without him does he recognize that his actions have made a difference. By the time the film ends, George has regained hope. He is able to face the threat of bankruptcy and prison gladly, secure in the knowledge that even such calamities cannot make his life worthless.

Art, it is said, imitates life. The themes that make *It's a Wonderful Life* so widely popular are not screenwriters' artifice; they are feelings that have their roots in the real world. I can't help but bring them to mind when I think about the epidemic of human immunodeficiency virus. When we visualize the end of the AIDS epidemic, we tend to think of a vaccine or a medical cure. We expect scientific experts to deliver us from this plague, to learn enough about the virus to beat it. As a society we have a sturdy confidence in the ability of science to improve our lives. But we can also look at the end of AIDS in a way that doesn't put all the responsibility into the hands of scientific experts. Truck drivers and working mothers, schoolchildren and bartenders also have the means to end this epidemic—not by studying molecular genetics or conducting clinical trials but through a shared resolve to become personally involved as individuals, families, and communities in preventing the spread of HIV.

Like Mr. Capra's critics, some readers may consider this notion too simplistic. They may think it reflects sentiment rather than science and promotes populism in place of public health policy. Truly, it will not be easy to stop AIDS. There are so many barriers to preventing HIV infection, both personal and social—discrimination, ignorance, inadequate resources, profound differences of perspective, to name a few. Still, effective tools and strategies are available to us if we are willing to use them: honest media campaigns promoting the use of condoms for sexually active people; school-based programs that teach children about human sexuality and provide them with the information and skills to make wise and healthy choices about sex; readily available treatment programs for people whose use of drugs puts them at continual risk for HIV infection; and sustained community programs in which ordinary people help their friends and neighbors, folks like themselves, to understand their risk of HIV infection and protect themselves against it. In order for these tools to be effective, however, we must be willing to accept as equivalent to our own the thoughts and feelings of people whose heritage, rearing, and life experiences may be profoundly different from ours. We must respond to the AIDS epidemic as a threat to humanity, not just as a problem of selected groups. Scientists and government officials cannot create this response, but ordinary people like George Bailey can.

The other element of Capra's film which viewers find so attractive is the conviction that people can overcome despair, that life provides second chances. In the film the mediator of this reprieve is a kindly, bumbling guardian angel. Who's to say if such amiable spirits exist? If they do, how often do they trouble themselves with the cares of this world? I don't know. But there have been people in my life, flesh-and-blood people, who have made a difference, who have given me second chances by helping me to appreciate life, just as surely as George's angel, Clarence, helped him.

Because of the people I loved who died of AIDS, I have had no need for a divinely staged version of "Had You Never Been Here," no need to turn back the clock, to subtract my presence from the events taking place around me.

Their suffering and death has been my version of Potters-
ville. Seeing their lives cut short, seeing them stumbling on
canes or confined to wheelchairs years before nature would
have required such accommodations, has been my personal
version of *It's a Wonderful Life.*

Remembrance

I shall remember while the light lives yet
And in the night time I shall not forget.

A. C. SWINBURNE
"Erotion"

SALVADOR DALI'S PAINTING *The Persistence of Memory* depicts a desolate landscape of desert and sea in which are arranged strange images of soft-boiled timepieces and incomplete forms only partially recognizable as human. I'm not sure that I understand everything the artist was trying to say about memory in that work, but I do agree with two of his points: that memory is plastic and that it is peculiar.

One of the reasons memories change is that we change. I don't just mean physiologically, though physiology is certainly a factor. Our life span is finite; the equipment isn't meant to last forever. Still, changes in our physical capacity to process, store, and resurrect memories may be less profound than the changes in perspective we experience as we pass through life. Part of what Dali says in his painting is that memories of past events are not fixed but fluid. They can be influenced by our experiences of the present.

Because of this uniquely human ability to reconfigure the past, to reinterpret it in the light of new experiences, remembrance is a powerful force in our lives. Memories are not musty parchment scrolls kept within an obscure cabinet on some inaccessible shelf. They are living documents, works that can be pulled down, reexamined, and edited in light of recent events.

The way I remember my friend Martin's death has changed over time. Shortly after his funeral, I could not get past the memory of his mother's tears and his waxen fingers—how he looked lying in the open coffin. Then, the reality of death was a new experience for me. Now, I am more likely to remember the last time I saw him alive. Two weeks before his death, I happened to be in town on business, and we'd arranged to have dinner together. He didn't tell me he was sick; in fact, he never told anyone. Only afterward did his friends and family learn he had AIDS. Several months had passed since I'd seen him last, and I could tell that he wasn't well, even though he brushed aside my questions about how he was feeling. He'd lost so much weight that his eyes seemed too large for his face.

I remember that he was very serious during our last meeting together—not morose, just intent on talking about things that would have been described as "heavy" when the two of us were in college together. He talked about making drastic changes in his life, about leaving his profession and abandoning the responsibilities of a regimented, demanding job. "Think about how great it would be," he said, "to buy an old trailer and travel around the country with a carnival—selling french fries and hot dogs." At the time his musings struck me as odd, even somewhat irresponsible. My profession has always been a source of self-esteem, and my work an important part of my life. I couldn't "get into" (another expression from our youth) the notion of tossing it aside. But I sat and listened. Mostly I nodded and let Martin go on. He'd manifested a strong hedonistic streak since our early college days. One of his intriguing qualities was his willingness to look for personal satisfaction, not in a cruel or careless way but as an honest and unashamed statement of his individual priorities.

Two weeks after that evening, when the phone rang at five o'clock in the morning and his mother told me Martin was dead, I remembered our dinner conversation. He was trying to tell me he was dying, I thought. He realized that everything was coming to an end, but he just didn't know how to tell me. That was why, I reasoned, he spoke of abandoning his job.

Lately I've been thinking that maybe I was wrong about the meaning of my last conversation with Martin. More and more I believe that what he was talking about that evening was living, not dying. Now, when I remember our dinner together, I think that he was trying to share a discovery with me, to pass along something important he'd learned from life. If we are not careful, he was telling me, the demands and obligations of our lives can crowd out our need for fulfillment. We should not think less of ourselves if our dreams and plans are different from what others expect them to be.

I still miss Martin; there is no one else like him. He was blessed with the capacity to find happiness in events and circumstances that to others would have seemed quite ordinary. If he had a sunny day and a full pack of Newports, he was ready to take on the world. I've never known anyone else who was so easily satisfied.

It's funny, but I can no longer visualize his face as it appeared in the casket. I remember so many things about that day: the large floppy bow on his sister's black dress, the yellow roses on the octagonal table in the foyer of the funeral home, and the stories and remembrances we shared as we sat next to the body of our friend. I know what his face looked like; I can describe it. I just can't see it. When I try to picture it now, I can only see Martin as he appeared when we were in college together, his eyes squeezed together tight and his mouth open wide in laughter.

Family Values

The hand that gives, gathers.

PROVERB

ACCORDING TO RICHARD LEAKEY, many of the characteristics that distinguish us from the other primates developed from our ancestors' practice of sharing food. In his book *Origins,* Leakey posits that collective participation in hunting and sharing of the quarry stimulated a social structure that was cooperative, mutually dependent, and self-trusting. Leaky points out that sharing on this scale is unique among primates; he believes that it stimulated the development of individual and group skills that were eventually responsible for the advancement of our species.

After a million or so years of existing as hunters and gatherers, about ten thousand years ago, according to Leakey, we humans tried our hand at organized agriculture. The growing of crops permitted the accumulation of a food surplus, which, in turn, supported population concentration and the development of the first cities. Prehistory soon became history.

The power of Leakey's hypothesis that our humanity derives from the act of sharing overwhelms me. I realize that people who make their living thinking and writing about evolution are more likely to describe this adaptation in functional rather than symbolic terms. They'd probably say

that those hominid packs that adopted the sharing behavior adapted better to their environment because they
were more efficient hunters; they prospered compared to
those groups that did not share. I also realize that Leakey's
isn't the only theory explaining how humans evolved from
the hominid herd. Nevertheless, his hypothesis seems to me
the grandest of metaphors for what it means to be human.
We became human by acting in human ways, and sharing
was the first truly human act.

Can a million-year-old social standard be relevant in
today's world? Our problems are more complex, our awareness of the ambiguous more profound. Some characteristics
of prehistoric society, such as division of labor on the basis
of sex, are now considered anathema by many modern *Homo
sapiens.* Is the act of sharing, in the way it was practiced by
our ancestors, still relevant to the way we live today?

Much as we might be tempted to romanticize sharing by
attributing it to altruistic motives, it was first and foremost
a practical adaptation. Our ancestors chanced upon the
discovery that the volume of flesh and the frequency of the
kill could be dramatically increased by employing group
rather than individual effort. The group didn't consist only
of those who tracked the beast or wielded the rocks. It also
included those who cooked and stored the flesh and tended
the young when the hunters were off pursuing game. To
ensure the viability of this arrangement, whose goal, after
all, was to procure food, each of the participants had to
receive a share of the spoils. If not, what would be the
motivation for cooperating? Food was shared because our
forebears came to recognize that the contributions of each
were critical to the success of the whole group; without
cooperation it was more difficult to assuage hunger. Look-

ing at it from a twentieth-century perspective, the needs of each member of the group were validated because each member contributed to group success.

A million years later, the quest to end hunger is only one of many pressing social goals. Would sharing, the prehistoric trait that first made us human, help us to meet these goals? I believe it would.

The prevention of HIV infection, for example, is a common social goal. Everyone supports it; we've had few problems recognizing that it's in our best interest to control the AIDS epidemic. But when we begin talking specifically about how to achieve this goal, the discussion often becomes divisive. We adopt one of two basic views: either we see HIV infection as a threat to *us*, to the members of *our* society, or we see people who are at risk for acquiring and transmitting HIV as outsiders.

When we look at HIV infection as a threat to our own, we accept as valid the prevention needs of those of us who are at risk, and we willingly share our resources to meet their needs. We don't limit our support to a litany of negatives: "stop using drugs," "stop being sexually attracted to persons of your own sex," or "stop thinking about having sexual intercourse; you're too young." Our ancestors might as well have said to their kin, "Stop thinking about meat and you won't be hungry." We accept what our fellow human beings tell us about the way they feel and think because we don't want to lose their social contributions; we cooperate with one another.

If we don't see those whose behaviors and circumstances place them at risk for HIV infection as part of our group, we are unlikely to see how their well-being and health contributes to our own, and we'll be less likely to consider their specific prevention needs as worthy of consuming limited societal resources. Consider the drug user whose practice of sharing needles puts him or her at ongoing risk for HIV infection. Do we consider the injecting drug user's need for drug treatment a high priority? And when some drug users tell us that they have no intention of stopping but want to limit their chances of getting AIDS by using clean needles, how seriously have we considered this request?

To be fair, modern humans find it more difficult to cooperate with one another, not because we've become more quarrelsome or less aware of the value of sharing. It's simply that it was much easier for our ancestors to understand how the person who threw the rock or skinned the carcass contributed to the good of the group than it is for us to appreciate how people who seem so different from us contribute to our own well-being. But if we stop to consider the loss of human potential and the other tremendous social costs associated with the HIV epidemic, we see how it is in everyone's interest to slow its spread.

Our world is defined by the people who live in it. How could it be otherwise? People who aren't all the same, who differ in color and sexual orientation and social circumstance, are part of our human race. If we refuse to listen to them, if we refuse to share societal resources to meet their expressed prevention needs, we will pay a price. We will lose something of what it means to be human.

My Father's Bakery

As you bake so shall you eat.

PROVERB

As someone who's been to more than one commencement exercise, I know it's flattering to think that a string of degrees behind one's name indicates wisdom and authoritative skill. But knowledge doesn't reside exclusively in classrooms, nor is it possessed solely by people with formal schooling. University professors weren't the only ones who taught me about medicine and public health. I also learned from sick and dying patients, from health workers who volunteered at a free clinic, from orderlies who'd never finished high school, even from people who weren't involved in the fields of medicine or public health at all. Long before I'd heard of the health consumerism movement or about the role of client preference in the design of health promotion programs, my father taught me that we must understand and respect the wishes of our customers if we expect to meet their needs.

I come from a family of bakers. Shortly after they arrived from Italy, my great-grandmother and her sons started their first American bakery in a small western Pennsylvania town called Belle Vernon. Those were the days when women either baked at home or purchased their bread in neighborhood shops. Supermarkets, with their mass-produced, gleaming white bread, were not yet a fixture of urban life.

The European immigrants who filled the hillside towns of the Monongahela River valley and worked in its glass factories, coal mines, and steel mills were good customers. Eventually, several of great-grandmother's sons, my grandfather included, opened their own bakeries. From the age of thirteen, my father learned about baking by working alongside his father. After my grandfather died, Dad started his own bakery.

Because my father's bakery was a family business, all of us worked there at one time or another. My father was both baker and business manager. My mother kept the books and supervised the women who worked as clerks. On Saturdays, my sister worked as one of the "store girls," and my brother and I scrubbed dirty pans. The summer after my first year of college, I worked as an apprentice to my father. In addition to learning how to roll pie crust—a skill I have retained ever since—I had an opportunity to observe the workings of my father's bakery at close range.

The life of a baker is harder than one might imagine. People tend to think of flour and icing, white aprons and meringue, which don't usually imply arduous labor, especially when compared to workplace images like axles and grease or the blistering heat of a Bessemer furnace. But do not be deceived. Hundred-pound sacks of flour are no lighter than hundred-pound pieces of scrap metal, and the heat of a bread oven on a summer morning can be stifling. Awakening before dawn six days a week so that the dough has time to rise and the ovens time to heat requires both discipline and a strong constitution.

In the microcosm of the bakery, as in society at large, a variety of skills are required to create and sell a successful product. Take birthday cakes as an example. Most of us bring to mind the final outcome: delicately scripted congratulations and brightly colored icing roses atop alternate layers of cake and filling. But making a successful birthday cake requires more than the skills of a good decorator. A number of people contribute to the effort: the clerk who takes the phone order, the flour salesperson who supplies the ingredients, the apprentice who combines them, the baker who makes sure that the cakes don't burn in the oven, and the helper who cleans the cake pans after the baking is finished. To the customer, these efforts are largely invisible, but anyone who has worked in a bakery knows that they are critical to customer satisfaction. After all, it doesn't matter how good a cake tastes or how pretty it looks if its salutation is addressed to the wrong person or if it's not ready on the day that it's needed. Above all else, my father worried about keeping his customers happy. He would repeat over and over to all of us his golden rule of consumer relations: "The customer is always right." On those rare occasions when a customer wasn't satisfied with a product, my father had instructed the "store girls" to listen politely and offer to replace the purchase immediately. There was to be no bickering, no challenge to the perceptions of the customer.

The importance of meeting consumer needs may not seem like a profound truth. Yet, these many years later, I am struck by its elemental relevance to the work of AIDS prevention. A large body of research both within and outside the AIDS arena consistently shows that programs to encourage healthier behavior are doomed to failure if they are not grounded on the needs and wants of the people for whom they are intended. In other words, products, whether chocolate chip cookies or AIDS-prevention services, are not made solely to serve the needs of the seller; they must also meet the needs of the buyer; otherwise, what's the basis for the exchange? Customers won't buy a product, even of

the highest quality, if it isn't something they want or perceive they need. When health-promotion efforts fail to
produce results, it is often because the architects of such
efforts have neglected, ignored, or misinterpreted the needs
of their customers. For example, many studies show that
female prostitutes who regularly use condoms during commercial acts of intercourse often do not use them with their
husbands or lovers. Frequently, this is because of their
perception that condoms interfere with sexual intimacy,
something that is very important to them in their primary
relationships. These women may also incorrectly gauge
their risk of acquiring HIV infection from their partners as
significantly less than it is from their clients—even though
their partners may be at high risk through unsafe practices
such as injecting drug use. When "selling" condom use as a
prevention strategy to women who trade sex for economic
purposes, AIDS educators must employ different counseling approaches for commercial and emotional sexual acts.

They say that people entering middle age are prone to
romanticize their youth. Perhaps I am no exception. When
I think back on that summer I spent in my father's bakery,
it seems that I learned so many lessons that are of value to
me today—that discipline, skill, and stamina are needed to
create something worthy from the raw and unfinished, that
doing a job well is rarely the result of one person working
alone, but more often of a team of people working together.
And I will never forget my father's exhortation that what is
most important about exchanges between a buyer and a
seller is what the consumer thinks about the product, not
what the seller thinks about the consumer.

I learned something else that summer I spent in the
bakery. Sometimes, no matter how well you scour the mix-
ing bowl before you whip the meringue, it just doesn't set

up. You don't know why; you just know that it hasn't. And even when there's water in the steam box and you've followed the recipe exactly, your bread dough may not rise the way it should. Perhaps it was the yeast, maybe the temperature. Baking, like life, can result in disappointment, even when you've played by the rules and followed the instructions carefully. The best you can do is try again until you get it right.

Once, during that summer, the timer on our big oven broke and an entire batch of egg custard pies was burned. My mother, who abhorred waste, fussed about the loss, wondering if there were some way to retrieve any of the pies. My father surveyed the damage. Around his eyes and mouth I could see the faintest trace of disappointment, but his voice was firm when he answered, "Throw them out." Within minutes he was back at the mixer, humming and joking with the other bakers as he began to combine fresh ingredients for a new batch of pies. They came out just fine.

The Language of Flowers

The morning glory which blooms for an hour
Differs not at heart from the giant pine
Which lives for a thousand years.

ZEN POEM

GARDENING ENCOMPASSES MORE than the physical chores of watering, weeding, and pruning; above all else, it is a commitment to nurture. Gardeners come to see the plants in their care as individual living entities, not just as adornments to the landscape. When they flourish, we applaud their success and should they succumb to blight, we regret their loss. For me, this close involvement with plants has resulted in occasional flights of fancy, during which I wonder what the plants in my garden would say if only they could talk to one another.

I suspect that, like humans, they would fall back on a number of standard topics of conversation. Some subjects, like the weather, would likely be even more popular in the plant kingdom than they are in the human realm; it's hard to imagine a garden plant not having an opinion on the prevailing climate. With the right amount of imagination, we could hear their whispery voices complaining about the weather, grumbling that it is too changeable—too wet one week, too dry the next. Lobelia, turtlehead, and marsh marigold, three sturdy plants that thrive near streams and in bogs, would be enthusiastic supporters of damp and drizzly days. Others, such as portulaca, finding the endless rain moldy and depressing, would long for days that are dry and lizard-hot, days when the sky is filled with nothing but the sun.

I imagine, too, that disease would be a frequent topic of conversation, since threats to well-being are never uninteresting to any living creature. Monarda and phlox would commiserate about their powdery mildew, each holding out its splotched leaves, like two veterans comparing battle scars, to see which of the two was more afflicted. They would lament that they aren't as hardy as rudbeckia, which never seems to be bothered by any blight or infestation. From closer to the ground, lamium would let out a squeaky protest that its misery from slugs was far worse than any powdery mildew. Many others would join in, the older asters sharing stories about seasons past when the blister beetles were so bad that only one of every ten buds actually bloomed. Suddenly, all would become quiet and begin nervously to inspect their stems and leaves for signs of insect infestation—except for the verbena, which talks on and on long after the others have become uncomfortable with the subject.

In my fantasy, there is more to the conversation of plants than drought, drench, and plague. Like us, they have their happy times too. For garden plants, few occasions are as joyous as the Day of First Blooming, when wilt and blight are not so much denied as ignored. Whereas on other days of the growing season plants might talk with regret about what could have been had they only had more rainfall and compost or fewer bugs to contend with, on this day all such talk is banished. The Day of First Blooming is not a time to offer excuses or to long for things that cannot be; it is a day to celebrate existence, aphids and all.

Even before the sun rises on that day, when the moon-light still colors the drops of dew on their leaves a milky blue, their excited whispers can be heard throughout the garden. From plant to plant they pass the news. "Did you hear that lychnis is going to bloom today?" The annuals, excited as children on Christmas Eve, titter among themselves until they are overheard by the shade perennials at the other end of the garden. Hosta is the first to get the news and spreads it quickly among the astilbes and to heuchera. By the time dawn breaks, all the perennials, most of the shrubs, and even a few of the more observant grasses have heard. And now they eagerly await the morning, their leaves and flower heads turned toward lychnis.

And what about lychnis, the object of every plant's interest and admiration? As the morning passes and the sun reaches toward noon, yesterday's swollen buds have opened, revealing deep magenta blooms held up by stalks of velvety silver. If we could only hear them, the herbs and ground-covers, the perennials and the shrubs, we would know that each one is murmuring, "Look at us. Look at us." There is nothing plaintive about their request. Soft as it is, it is none-theless joyful. For knowledge of the coming frost is not a cause for despair, but a reason to cherish blooming.

Gardening in Clay

Not in the clamour of the crowded street,
Not in the shouts and plaudits of the throng,
But in ourselves, are triumph and defeat.

HENRY WADSWORTH LONGFELLOW
"The Poets"

ALL NORMAL SOILS are made up of five components in various combinations: mineral fragments from rock, decaying organic matter, living organisms, air, and water. The soils that result from different combinations of these five elements wield a profound influence over whether plants will flourish or perish after a period of half-hearted growth.

Soils are further categorized by their consistency. Sandy soils have the largest particles and clay soils the smallest, with silt soils falling in between. Successful garden soil should be a balanced combination of clay, silt, humus, and sand. The balance is quite important. Too much clay and the soil will be soggy and poorly aerated. Too much sand and it will fail to hold moisture and mineral elements long enough for the plants to take advantage of them. Not enough humus and the soil will be poor in texture and bereft of organic nutrients.

Those who have gardened in clay soil, as I have, know these facts to be true from bitter and disappointing experi-

ence. At my home in Atlanta, I have a garden bed in which
the soil is terrible—just solid clay. At first, I underestimated
the importance of this fact. I had expected the soil of the
south to be different from the rich loam of western Pennsylvania, where I was raised. I had anticipated the red color
and I thought that the thick and lumpy consistency must
just be the way southern soil feels. And besides, the clay
didn't seem to stunt the growth of the unwieldy ligustrum
that I had to clear to make space for my flower bed. Then
too, I was impatient. In my mind's eye my garden had already reached maturity, and I pictured abundant color and
form, flowers of all types. I reasoned that with diligent
care on my part, close attention to weed control and plenty
of water during those hot summer months, I could overcome any soil imperfections. I planted a number of annuals
and perennials in informal groupings within the space I'd
cleared, certain that by midsummer there would be glorious
results.

But it didn't work that way. At least not in the time
frame I had imagined. The first to go were the dusty millers.
Throughout the spring, they seemed to grow more slowly
than I thought they should, and early in the summer their
fine silver leaves became bloated and dull. Eventually, all but
a few withered and died. Seeing such a common plant fail to
grow filled me with a dread that others would soon follow. I
was not long in waiting.

The ageratums, which had always reminded me of my
Aunt Rose's summer garden, were the next to succumb. The
casual mounds of fluffy blue flowers that I remembered so
well from my childhood had little in common with the
puny and frail productions of these plants. So many plants
perished that first growing season—coreopsis, gaillardia,

yarrow, and foxglove. Some managed to produce a few mealy blooms; others didn't achieve even that meager success.

After so much death and disappointment, I decided it was time for action. I had made a grave mistake in minimizing the significance of something as fundamentally important as soil quality, but there were ways that it could be improved, and I intended to employ them. I was determined that my garden match the image I had nurtured in my mind. I wanted to be able to smell and touch those mounds of color, to see the blossoms pressed down heavily after a summer rainstorm, to spread their fragrance around my house in vases and glasses and jars. I was willing to accept some disease and death, every gardener must, but not on such a large and relentless scale.

And so it began. That fall and each one since, I have added the elements that were lacking to my garden soil. Peat moss and leaf mulch to improve the soil texture and to provide the missing organic nutrients. Sharp, angular sand, not the smooth kind found in children's playboxes, to increase the soil particle size so that the roots would have an easier time in their search for water and oxygen. And composted cow manure and granular fertilizers as additional enrichments.

Each growing season since, I have seen an improvement in my plants. They haven't yet matched the ideal in my mind, but they come closer and closer every year. The delicate ones have been slower to take hold, but the sturdy perennials, such as aster, rudbeckia and echinacea, are doing just fine. Although I enjoy picking great bunches of them to place around the house in late summer, that is not the most gratifying time for me as a gardener. No, the best time for me is each fall when I haul the sacks of sand and peat and manure from the nursery to my backyard and work them, with spade and shovel, into the soil. For me it's a time for remembering those first plantings that ended so poorly. It may seem a foolish reverie, but when I'm turning up the soil and breaking apart the lumps of clay I still occasionally encounter, I think about those first plants as heroes. Their death helped me improve as a gardener, just as surely as any book or newspaper column on gardening. As I work the soil, sometimes with my bare hands, I am filled with anticipation for what the spring will bring. I know that with each season the soil will continue to improve and more plants will flourish until finally even the most tender perennials will thrive in what was once a sodden and hopeless plot of clay.